D0614636

The Successful
Caregiver's Guide

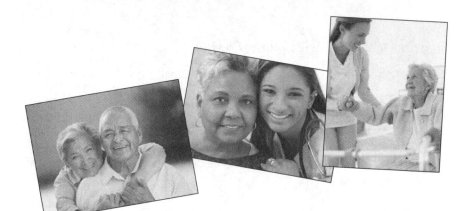

The Successful
Caregiver's Guide

Rick Lauber

Self-Counsel Press Inc.
(a subsidiary of)
International Self-Counsel Press Ltd.
USA   Canada

Copyright © 2015 by Self-Counsel Press Inc.

All rights reserved.

No part of this book may be reproduced or transmitted in any form by any means — graphic, electronic, or mechanical — without permission in writing from the publisher, except by a reviewer who may quote brief passages in a review.

Printed in Canada.

First edition: 2015

Library of Congress Control Number: 2015936847

Self-Counsel Press Inc.
(a subsidiary of)
International Self-Counsel Press Ltd.

Bellingham, WA
USA

North Vancouver, BC
Canada

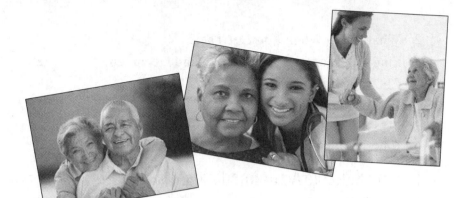

Contents

13 Finding Joy in Caregiving

14 Final Thoughts

Download kit

Worksheets

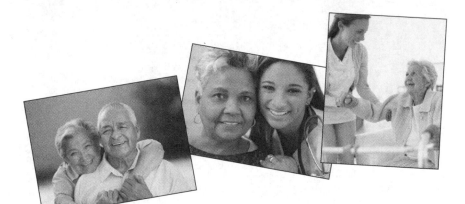

Notice to Readers

Laws are constantly changing. Every effort is made to keep this publication as current as possible. However, the author, the publisher, and the vendor of this book make no representations or warranties regarding the outcome or the use to which the information in this book is put and are not assuming any liability for any claims, losses, or damages arising out of the use of this book. The reader should not rely on the author or the publisher of this book for any professional advice. Please be sure that you have the most recent edition.

Website links often expire or web pages move, at the time of this book's publication the links were current.

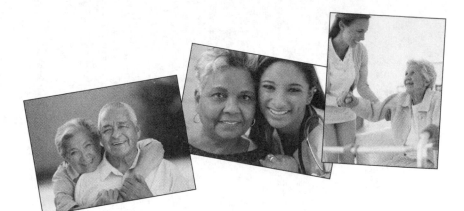

Acknowledgments

In memory of Mom and Dad.

With appreciation to Susan and Barb for their invaluable help with the "Aged Ps."

Thanks to Chris for her love, patience, support, and understanding while I wrote this book.

In recognition of all who selflessly provide formal or informal care at any level.

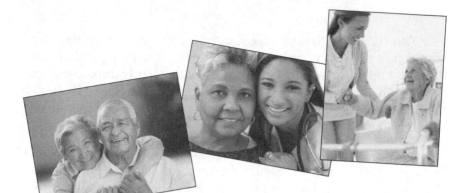

Introduction

Residents of the United States have weathered hurricanes (e.g., Galveston, Texas, 1900; and Hurricane Katrina, 2005), faced fires (e.g., Yarnell Hill Fire, Prescott, Arizona, 2013), and coped after world terrorism (911, New York City, 2001). After each catastrophe, Americans have proven themselves to be admirably resilient by surviving and rebuilding. However, there is a brewing problem throughout the country and it requires immediate attention: The country's aging population. As of 2010, 40.3 million seniors (those 65 and older) were living in the United States — a notable jump of 15.1 percent of the country's population between 2000 and 2010.[1]

With aging baby boomers (defined by the US Census Bureau as children born between 1946 and 1964 and directly following World War II), these numbers will most certainly increase. More and more adult children will see their own parents age and decline due to physical or mental health issues. As parents age, many sons and daughters will become caregivers who will help and support their aging parents in any number of ways. While aging, sickness, and eventual death are not pleasant topics to think or talk about, denial of these facts is not an answer. Mom or Dad may seem fine today, but she or he could easily fall and break a hip tomorrow. Realistically, one must expect and prepare for the future caregiving role.

---

1 "65+ in the United States: 2010," Loraine A. West, Samantha Cole, Daniel Goodkind, and Wan He; United States Census Bureau; accessed April 2015. https://www.google.ca/?gws_rd=ssl#q=2010%2C+40.3+-million+seniors+%28those+older+than+65%29+were+living+in+the+United+States — a+notable+jump+of+15.1+percent+of+the+country%E2%80%99s+population+between+2000+and+2010

With the population of the United States rapidly aging, more adult children are scrambling to find and provide help for their own parents. Unless those family members have been fortunate enough to work in the health-care, financial, legal, or social-work fields, they often lack the necessary skills, attitudes, and experience to adequately help.

When it comes to caregiving, there is a huge sense of responsibility, obligation, and even guilt for these adult children who may silently believe, "Mom and Dad cared for me; now it's my turn." In turning the tables, adult children do what they can but must frequently learn "on the job" while giving their parents the best quality of life possible. (My decision to write this book was prompted by this very situation.) Often, there is not much time allowed for a caregiver to research an issue, deliberate with other family members, and/or reach a decision as to what to do. Commonly, family members serving as caregivers suffer from a sense of imbalance, stress, and myriad emotions that include anger, depression, confusion, and grief. Considering the consequences, this is not always best for either the family caregivers or their parents.

Whether you are becoming a caregiver, anticipating eventually taking on the role, currently providing parental care, or know of someone else wearing the caregiver's shoes, you are likely entering into foreign territory. There is no road map or tour guide to steer you in exactly the right direction. As a caregiver, you will be called on to make difficult lifestyle, health-care, and financial decisions affecting your own parents. You will struggle and question yourself as to whether you made the right and/or best choices. Learn to accept your own decisions, your own shortcomings (you cannot do it all for your parent), and the crucial importance of personal respite (i.e., taking a personal break).

Trust me, this is not easy. I've served as a caregiver not once, but twice — for both of my aging parents. My Mom had Parkinson's disease and Leukemia while Dad developed Alzheimer's disease. With Mom and Dad becoming sick simultaneously, my caregiving duties doubled and there was no rest between them. Through my experiences, I have developed a newfound respect for those working in care; specifically, for untrained family members (like me) who, often, have been thrust unknowingly and unprepared into a caregiving role. I have also gained more respect for myself and know my own strengths and weaknesses far better, as well as when it is necessary to take a break.

As you look ahead with uncertainty or trepidation to provide elder care, know that this is not a typical self-help book which simply aims to encourage or inspire you to learn something new or change your own life for the better. The issues I speak of in this book are very real, and the tools and strategies I suggest can be very effective. I will share stories with you as to what caregiving mechanisms were helpful for me, and I will also discuss what was not helpful.

For the sake of conciseness, I have chosen to remember my Dad for the most part throughout this book. While my Mom's medical case certainly presented numerous challenges, my Dad outlived her and my caregiving responsibilities were extended. Not all of this may be exactly relevant to your own situation, but please glean what you can from it. It is my hope that when you have finished reading this book, you will have learned at least one new thing about what to expect or how to cope as a caregiver.

There are stories of confusion, worry, and neglect that surround the role of caregiving. These stories greatly sadden me, but I would like to emphasize that caregiving is not all doom and gloom or death and despair. While your parent's situation (and perhaps your own) may seem bleak to you, there is great joy to be found here as you will see in the following pages.

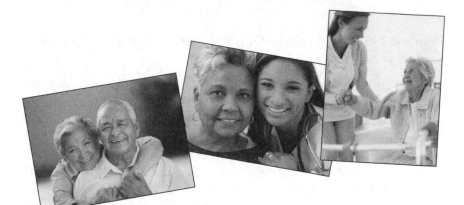

Chapter 1
Defining Caregiving

"One person caring about another represents life's greatest value."

– Jim Rohn

It's interesting (and somewhat unsettling) that, while the word "caregiving" is becoming much more used these days, the term remains largely misunderstood. There could be any number of reasons why including a lack of understanding about the job, a feeling of shame or discomfort (people may not readily admit they are doing this), or a sense of obligation (since Mom or Dad took care of me, it's now my turn to care for them).

A friend of mine explained that she routinely visits a blind woman to open and read her mail. When I immediately defined my friend as a "caregiver" she hesitated initially, but soon admitted that she was indeed providing care and support — what she was doing was an important task — albeit on a smaller scale than what others might do.

While many have chosen to ignore or completely dismiss the impact of caregiving on others, the facts point to this as an ever-growing problem and growth trend. Undeniably, the United States has a graying population. The children of World War II (those born between

1946 and 1964) are growing older. These are society's baby boomers; I'm in this category myself.

According to the Family Caregiver Alliance, "65.7 million caregivers make up 29% of the US adult population providing care to someone who is ill, disabled, or aged."[1] You don't have to look too far to find other statistics echoing this magnitude. The Alzheimer's Association reports that "43.5 million of adult family caregivers care for someone 50+ years of age and 14.9 million care for someone who has Alzheimer's disease or other dementia."[2] The United States Census reveals that the country had 40.3 million people 65 or older in 2010 — the highest number of seniors since the Census Bureau began keeping records more than a century ago. Not surprisingly, California is the state with the largest number of residents 65 and older with 4.2 million; followed by Florida with 3.3 million; New York and Texas are tied with 2.6 million; and Pennsylvania with 2 million.

These numbers are certainly not stagnant. They are, in fact, expected to skyrocket. By 2035, the country's 65-plus population is expected to more than double. While this will be good news for those in senior-serving professions (as it results in more work and more opportunities), it will result in many more family members stepping forward to provide care for loved ones. Without proper preparation and education, these family members will be caught improvising and struggling (as I did).

A high population of seniors is not just an American issue; it is fast becoming a global concern. Caregiving does not have any borders. In Canada, almost 15 percent of the country's population is now aged 65 years or older. According to the International Alliance of Carer Organizations, there were 6.5 million caregivers in the UK (2009), 1.3 million caregivers (aged 18+) in Sweden (2012), and 2,694,600 caregivers in Australia (2012).[3] Another report from the National Bureau of Statistics of China noted that the number of people, nationwide aged 60 years and older reached 167 million (or 12.5 percent of the total population) in 2009.[4]

Should these numbers not speak to you, know that aging is a natural course of life and a high population of seniors is almost guaranteed

---

1 "Caregiving in the US National Alliance for Caregiving Washington, DC," The National Alliance for Caregiving and AARP (updated November 2012).
2 "2011 Alzheimer's Disease Facts and Figures," Alzheimer's and Dementia, Volume 7, Issue 2; Alzheimer's Association (updated November 2012).
3 "Caregiving Statistics by Nation," International Alliance of Carer Organizations (IAC), accessed April 2015. http://www.caregiving.org/wp-content/uploads/2010/11/Caregiving-Statistics-by-Nation.pdf.
4 "The Old in China Have No Place to Live," Sify News, accessed April 2015. http://www.sify.com/news/the-old-in-china-have-no-place-to-live-news-international-kk0n4lgddfd.html

as baby boomers age. This is an oncoming speeding train that cannot be avoided. We can neither jump out of the way of nor blindly ignore this problem. With the rise of seniors expected, there will also be a correlating rise in the number of professional and private caregivers.

1. The Different Types of Caregivers

A caregiver can be simply defined as anyone who helps with the needs of others impacted by disease, disability, or aging. It's important to realize that caregivers exist on many different levels. There are, of course, the medical doctors who practice full-time, the nurses who travel from hospital room to hospital room, and the volunteers who push around patients in wheelchairs. A caregiver may also work part time and may not even identify as someone caring for another. A neighbor could mow the lawn or shovel the snow for a house-bound senior, a friend could drop in for a coffee and a chat, or an adult child could prepare and deliver a home-cooked meal. A minister can provide care on a spiritual level. A musician can visit a long-term care center and entertain residents with songs. No matter what level a person serves as a caregiver, he or she is doing noble work.

Caregivers are most often identified as adult children caring for aging parents; however, caregivers can be anyone. The list can include friends, spouses, partners, parents, and even grandparents. Care can be provided at many levels. In my friend's case, she reads a blind woman's mail; however, a caregiver can visit with a senior, provide transportation to medical appointments, serve as an advocate, manage finances, and help with hands-on care (e.g., clothing, toileting, or bathing). The list of caregiving jobs can seem endless and is rarely routine from one day to the next.

While caregivers may be handling tasks previously unknown to them, it's important for them to keep in their own comfort zones. I never helped my parents with bathing or showering, I felt this was better left to professionals who had more experience in this and knew how to keep a senior safe on a wet bathroom floor. The last thing I wanted to have happen is Mom or Dad falling as a result of my own inexperience in this area. The same can be said for physically lifting or transferring a senior. Doing this requires a certain procedure and expertise, and I knew full well that I was not the best person for this job.

Even young children can help to provide care. While they may not completely understand a senior's medical condition, young children can bring great joy and a breath of fresh air to a senior, so invite them along on visits. **Note:** When explaining the situation to children, it is important that they understand whatever ailment has been diagnosed is not anybody's fault and not contagious.

We often think of parents providing care for their own children. This is one of those most obvious examples of caregiving. With the United States' aging population, we are rethinking that norm and now understand and accept that adult children can easily become caregivers for their own parents.

Caregiving can inch up on you (e.g., a parent's chronic health condition) or it may happen overnight (e.g., a parent falls and as a result, becomes disabled). You can never forecast the future. For example, my father was always a little forgetful, so Alzheimer's disease was not a total surprise. My mother's conditions, conversely, came without any warning.

Other unexpected caregivers are not even human. Many seniors' homes are providing residents dogs or cats for "pet therapy." There is something very comforting and soothing about petting a dog or having a cat sitting on your lap. If you want to bring in the family dog or cat, please check with the care facility staff first. Depending on the size of the animal, it may startle or scare other residents. The best type of pet to bring will be one that is tame, quiet, and gentle around other people. Consider also that the sudden excited barking of a dog could upset other residents, and the cat could cause unpleasant and potentially dangerous allergic reactions for others. My parent's first residence when they returned to Edmonton was home to two colorful budgies. Mom and Dad, along with other residents in the building, found comfort and enjoyment watching and listening to the birds.

Caregivers can also be differentiated by being described as formal or informal caregivers. The "formal" group are often healthcare professionals who work in a related field. "Informal" caregivers are those family members who have little or no related experience and don't know what to expect. Formal and informal caregivers also have been categorized as "paid" and "unpaid." Family caregivers can, however, receive some kind of financial stipend paid from the parental bank account, should other family members agree.

No matter what type of health condition exists (e.g., cancer, multiple sclerosis, kidney disease), caregivers can face a steep, and often sudden, learning curve to become more knowledgeable. They will need to research the condition to become more knowledgeable with the symptoms, outcomes, and possible treatments.

Sometimes, family caregivers feel shame about having to care for aging parents. Feared humiliation or a lack of understanding from other individuals can lead to silence or reluctant whispers of admission. This is most unfortunate as caregivers should be proud of their role. By speaking out, caregivers may also find others willing and able to help them.

2. What Type of Caregiver Are You?

When it comes to caregiving categories, there are numerous types. There are many people who do not simply and neatly slide into one such category. Instead, they will show interest in a number of different areas and display different character traits. The trick is to know what you are best at and proceed accordingly.

It is perfectly natural to feel uncomfortable performing certain tasks for your loved one. Caregiving is often new ground for family members and it's not easy to watch Mom or Dad weaken without being able to do anything about it.

With the many unique situations and circumstances, I highly doubt I could ever create a universal template that all caregivers could follow. Resources, such as this book, can provide guidance and support; what your experience will become is yours and yours alone. However, you may find some similar experiences when sharing your situation with other caregivers.

People vary considerably with personalities, characters, abilities, mannerisms, and beliefs. What is "right" or proper for one person may not be so for another. Recognize your own strengths and weaknesses. As a new or current caregiver, you will need to consider (and continually consider) the following questions:

- What can you do?
- How much can you do?
- Is it important for you to manage specific issues and tasks?
- What do you want to do?
- How do you want to accomplish this?

- Who can help you?
- Can you work well with others or do you prefer to work independently?
- Can you lessen your load and delegate work to others?
- How would others describe you?

In business, entrepreneurs often conduct a preliminary "SWOT Analysis" to identify their strengths, weaknesses, opportunities, and threats in a business plan prior to opening shop. When pinpointing weaker areas of interest or capability in this manner, an entrepreneur will turn to a partner or an outside consultant for advice. Caregivers can follow suit here. By understanding your caregiving style, abilities, preferences, and physical location, you will be far better prepared to tackle tasks that come your way, and decide whether you want to leave them or delegate the jobs to someone else (who may be more willing and capable of doing the work than you). How you approach your own caregiving role is always your own way, so don't let anyone tell you what is best for you and your loved one. Grab a pen and paper because it's time to focus on you and to do an honest self-evaluation to identify your own caregiving characteristics.

If you don't know where to start, please refer to Worksheet 1: Caregiving Self-Analysis to help you identify your own strengths and weaknesses as a caregiver. (All worksheets in this book are also included in the download kit.)

Various caregiving characteristics are described by Shayne Fitz-Coy in his informative blog post, "Finding Your Caregiving Style."[5] The following sections cover my own experience as a caregiver, which is a variation on Fitz-Coy's listed characteristics.

You will likely recognize yourself as one, or even a combination of, the following caregiving types. As you will see, there is no cookie-cutter caregiver. You may fit neatly into one category or identify with many different caregiver traits. To be effective and successful with caregiving, you need to know what you are best at and proceed accordingly.

2.1 Independent caregiver

Are you determined, motivated, and stubborn? Do you want to tackle everything independently, and/or doubt that no one else could do

---

5 "Finding Your Caregiving Style," Shayne Fitz-Coy, Alert1 Medical Alert Systems, accessed April 2015. https://www.alert-1.com/blog/family-caregivers/finding-your-caregiving-style/1799

Worksheet 1
Caregiving Self-Analysis

Self-evaluation is crucial to caregivers. While you will be presented with many new responsibilities and challenges, you must know what you can do and the extent of your own personal limits.

Answer the following questions as honestly as you can. Addressing these issues sooner rather than later will help you identify your own strengths and weaknesses, which will be beneficial to you as a caregiver. Share these questions (and your answers, if you feel comfortable) with your siblings and delegate your roles appropriately.

1. What can you do as a caregiver?

2. How do you feel about becoming and acting as a caregiver?

3. What would you identify as your characteristic strengths and weaknesses?

4. Who will help you with your caregiving responsibilities? (Identify what others can do.)

5. Beyond your immediate circle of contacts, where will you look for additional help?

6. Can you work easily with others or do you prefer to work independently?

7. Are you flexible with your own schedule?

8. What negative issues do you foresee with serving as a caregiver?

9. How will you respond to or counteract these negative issues?

10. Where will you seek respite for your loved one?

11. Where will you seek respite for yourself?

12. List three additional ideas for personal coping and caring mechanisms (these will be new areas of interest to you that you could try in the future).

13. How much personal respite time will you give yourself?

14. What do you want to achieve as a caregiver?

15. Are you hesitant or reluctant to serve as a caregiver? If so, why?

16. How much will this hesitation interfere with your caregiving duties?

17. Will you be able to perform certain tasks or do you need to assign them to others?

18. Can you honestly look at yourself in the mirror and say, "I am doing the best job I can as a caregiver"?

19. Do you have any regrets about serving as a caregiver? If so, what are your regrets and how can you resolve them?

20. Where can you learn more about your loved one's medical condition and prognosis?

21. What other personal or professional demands, besides caregiving, exist for you?

22. How will you know you have done your best being a caregiver?

23. Are you an optimist or a pessimist? (Note that optimists will have an easier time and might be better caregivers.)

◇◇

the job better than you can? Do you feel resistance to sharing the work? These are not necessarily negative character traits.

The so-called independent caregivers may feel, and appear, confident and in total control with handling all the important affairs. The truth of the matter is, independent caregivers will be stretched to their very limits and must become even more flexible with balancing their time and lives. Independent caregivers, more so than other types of caregivers, can be called on at a moment's notice. Only adult children, by their very situations, will be tempted to be independent caregivers; however, it is even more vital for them to seek and secure the help of others.

2.2 Sharing caregiver

If you are able to collaborate, are able to balance the responsibilities or your own life and those of caregiving, and are team-oriented, then you may be a sharing caregiver. This caregiving arrangement requires partnering, working together, and compromising, so it helps considerably when siblings are on friendly terms. Having another family member (or two) available to handle what needs to get done increases balance and is more advantageous for all parties involved. It's always easier to carry a heavy load with assistance. This works best if the family members live relatively close to each other and the parent.

My older sister and I live in the same city (where Dad lived as well), my younger sister lives three hours south of us. Traveling, when required, was not impossible for my younger sister, but it could become very costly and inconvenient.

Realistically, you cannot expect a sibling to drive several hours into town at a moment's notice just to transport your parent to the doctor, pick up required medications, help tend to other needs, and allow you respite time. Considering the increased distance, further planning and coordinating of schedules may be required. Instead, explore other options of how that sibling living further away can help. The problem, however, is the sibling living closest to a parent often may be shouldered with all the necessary errands (simply due to convenience). If this occurs, then this individual should be compensated in some manner (e.g., a regular top up of gas for his or her vehicle would be greatly appreciated and shouldn't be a difficult decision for other family members to agree on). Your parent may require more immediate treatment that cannot wait.

2.3 Collaborative caregiver

A collaborative caregiver is practical, sensible, realistic, and resourceful. Consider yourself very lucky if you fall into this category. Similar to a sharing caregiver, a collaborative caregiver will participate as a caregiver; however, he or she will have the necessary resources to call on many others to provide proper care. This is one of the best approaches with elder care as it is not a job to undertake independently.

Take a few moments to identify these individuals and outside services by using Worksheet 2: Your Circle of Caregiving. Think outside the box here and include individuals, groups, and services. For example, collaborative caregivers may rely on nursing staff at a long-term care facility, a private companion, an activity coordinator who plans specialized outings for seniors, or a respite group that takes the parent for the day.

As the old saying goes, "Many hands make light work." As a collaborative caregiver, you will find you can better handle what is required and benefit from some regular time yourself. If you are not a collaborative caregiver, try becoming more of one. Doing so is certainly advantageous because it will benefit your own physical and mental health. Your own workload will be reduced resulting in your not being as busy or emotionally taxed. Such an arrangement works well to help you ease your stress.

2.4 Coordinating caregiver

Are you the type of person who researches, analyzes, and organizes everything? Have you been known to compare vacation destinations and flight schedules then create a to-do list of tasks and items to pack? This means you fall into the category of the coordinating caregiver.

Worksheet 2
Your Circle of Caregiving

As a caregiver, you can surround yourself with outside resources. Take some time to identify family, friends, colleagues, associations, seniors' programs, and seniors' services that can help you. It's not necessary to complete this worksheet in one sitting; you will add more names to your circle as you proceed. These will be new people you meet and helpful organizations. Having more helping hands involved with your parent's care will, ultimately, help you as a caregiver.

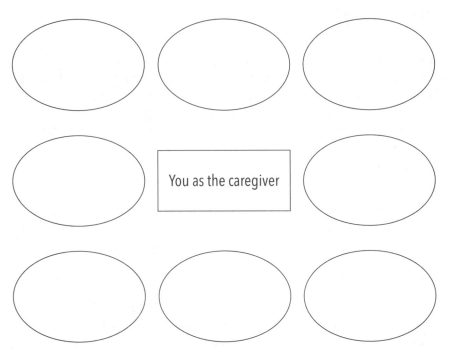

You will spend much of your time learning about relevant matters and then deciding on the best course of action. You will collect data and compare options such as researching medical advances, learning the possible side effects of prescribed medication, visiting long-term care facilities and assessing their suitability, or evaluating different models of motorized scooters.

You may have (perhaps color-coded) files for everything, you will keep brochures together, and you will remember to take receipts out of your shirt pockets before laundering. (That's the voice of experience speaking; I have routinely discovered wet and torn pieces of note paper in the washing machine after doing a load of laundry!)

As I've been known to scribble things down on spare pieces of paper and promptly lose those notes, I would not make an effective coordinating caregiver. This type of caregiver is highly organized.

2.5 Delegating caregiver

The delegating caregiver is the type of person who is dynamic, confident, and a leader (think of any past or present American president as a good example). This individual is the least hands-on because he or she assigns or hires people to provide the necessary care. Bringing in someone else for support isn't a bad thing at all; you may be uncomfortable with the necessary tasks or realize that others are infinitely more qualified (or have more time) to do some work than you are.

As for me, I see myself as a delegate caregiver as my professional background does not include anything resembling health care. I shied away from certain tasks and still feel to this day that assigning such responsibilities to me would have been both inappropriate and unsafe for my parents. While taking care of my parents was my responsibility, I realized that others could be involved so I utilized them.

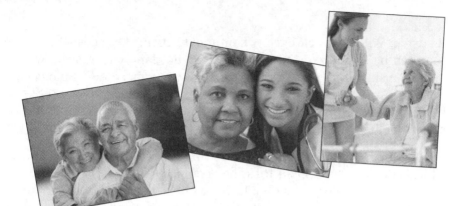

Chapter 2
Caring from a Distance

"You give but little when you give of your possessions.
It is when you give of yourself that you truly give."

– Kahlil Gibran

Families often drift apart geographically, which can make caregiving much more difficult. An outstretched hand can only reach so far. While caregiving from afar is certainly possible, it can be expensive and distant caregivers can pay the price in many ways.

I like to define a "long-distance caregiver" as someone who lives further than a one-hour drive from his or her aging parents. Realize that this hour is doubled to account for the return trip home and two hours on the road is almost 10 percent of a day. Long-distance caregivers are far more likely to miss full work days rather than caregivers living in the same neighborhood as their parents. This leads to long-distance caregivers spending more money (through lost income from missed work and higher costs involved to travel) than those who live closer to their parents.

Family caregivers can be caught between a rock and a hard place. Unfortunately, in our society, caregivers aren't often financially compensated leaving them paying out-of-pocket for expenses incurred. Will family caregivers continue to cover these costs? Until they can be subsidized for the work they do, family caregivers will be responsible for the costs. This, of course, can become a financial burden for many families. If a parent was financially savvy and has banked some savings, this can help, but, unfortunately, this does not always happen.

Warmer temperatures, like those in California, Arizona, and Florida, have great appeal for older people. Rural life can also be attractive for seniors. Smaller towns offer a more relaxed way of life with a close-knit community feel; yet, they can fall short when it comes to necessary care and resources. The nearest doctor's office may be located many miles away. The local hospital may not be prepared for all medical emergencies.

In my case, my parents retired from their previous, often chilly, family home where they had lived for 25 years to the much warmer clime of Victoria, British Columbia. I can't say that I blamed them for wanting to move there; however, my sisters and I quickly realized that Mom and Dad did not have much personal or professional support in their new home. This became painfully obvious when Mom needed immediate medical care. With her low hemoglobin counts, Mom was urged by her doctor to check into the hospital. Reportedly, Mom struggled physically to reach the hospital — stumbling down the street and often clasping on to street lamps for support.

My sisters and I were completely blind to all of this until my younger sister got a phone call from a social worker at the Victoria hospital. Mom, bless her soul, was concerned about leaving Dad alone at home. After a quick sibling discussion, we chose my younger sister as the most available to immediately fly to the island and help tend to Mom and Dad's needs. Fortunately for us, my younger sister's schedule allowed her some flexibility to do this. You may not be as lucky. You may be leading an important team project at work with a pressing deadline, your employer may be resistant about giving you time off on short notice, or you may have your own family obligations.

1. The Challenges of Long-Distance Caregiving

Caregiving, at any geographical distance, can be taxing; I found that long-distance caregiving increases the number of challenges. Most prevalent are the financial costs (e.g., long-distance phone calls and traveling expenses) which can easily skyrocket for distant family members. Frequently, caregivers pay for these expenses themselves — doing so can regrettably lead to resentment towards parents, the situation, and other siblings who may be blamed for not fully carrying their weight. Finding the best ways to say money and time may help reduce the resentment.

1.1 Communication

Even from a distance, communication is very possible. The telephone, fax, and postal services are old familiar standbys, but also consider the Internet. If your parents are tech-savvy, you can set up a web cam or buy a computer with one installed. With this, you can speak to and see your loved ones in real time. An email can be composed, sent, and received within mere minutes. Relevant website links, detailing important health information or otherwise, can be shared. You can also easily forward digital family photos. Pictures can be snapped, transformed into computer files, and sent electronically. Digitized information can be sent from you to your parents but also between you and your other siblings. A weekly email report summarizing your parent's latest news (health or otherwise) can be sent to brothers and/or sisters who live elsewhere. If you're in a time crunch, even a quick text message can be comforting and often enough to keep other family members involved.

Something you may want to consider is Skype, which is a computer program where you can call, video call, and instant message each other for free. You may also be familiar with FaceTime — the Apple version of this program. Note that as with anything new, your loved one must be comfortable using technology. Unfortunately, many seniors resist learning about (and utilizing) computers due to uncertainty, rigidity, or fear. Know and respect your parent's limits. Keep in mind, too, your parent's limiting factors — although my father had relied on a computer for his work for many years, Alzheimer's robbed him of his memories as to how to operate one (or even where to find the power button to turn on the machine).

When considering long-distance phone calls, limiting your calls to off-peak hours (when long-distance charges will be less) may seem easy enough; however, this cannot always happen. Many of the businesses, service centers, and doctors' offices that you will need to contact may not be open past 5:00 p.m. or on the weekends. When it comes to caregiving, you can never guarantee that your phone calls will only be required on evenings or weekends or at your own convenience. As a caregiver, you may be operating around the clock; however, business owners do not always recognize this same need.

A mobile phone, despite additional airtime charges, does have a distinct advantage for a caregiver. I am speaking of the added portability and convenience; you can carry a cell phone with you and place a call or receive a call almost anywhere. When I used my cell phone for such purposes, I referred to it as my "caregiving hotline" as I could be immediately reached.

With my mobile phone, I was offered the often-standard "free evenings and weekends" feature. I could make local calls between 5:00 p.m. and 6:00 a.m., Monday to Friday as well as all day on Saturday and Sunday, at no additional charge. Of the numerous airtime packages available, I then chose a basic deal for cost-savings. If you use more airtime minutes than what is agreed to in your sales contract, you will pay a cost per minute or per second. Be careful of this clause — should you talk for one minute and 15 seconds extra, you could be charged for two minutes.

I recommend that you shop around for a cell phone. Compare the look of the phone, the user-friendliness (are the buttons large enough for you to push?), and the offered deals. With airtime plans varying dramatically, consider them all carefully and ask yourself what works best for you. Think about your own cell phone usage: Will you really need 500-plus free daytime minutes on a monthly basis? That extra time will come at an extra price on your monthly bill. The good thing here is that there is some flexibility with airtime packages; you can always talk to your service provider about increasing or decreasing your allowed airtime.

My cell phone included a few additional features, which I found very handy when serving as a caregiver. Consider the following options. With voicemail, callers can leave a message. Although you can be more accessible with a cell phone, you may not always be available to take a call (e.g., many doctor's offices require patients to turn off their cell phones while inside). Call display shows the incoming caller's name and phone number. If I was busy with Mom or Dad when a call came through, I could quickly glance at my phone and decide whether to answer it or let it go through to voicemail. Call forwarding transfers incoming calls from one number to another. This feature I found repeatedly useful as people could still reach me when they only had my home number and I was away from home. Know that these little "extras" do cost more; however, they can be well worth it. On a related note, another practical tool is a car-charging cord for your cell phone; with this you may recharge a dwindling phone battery even when you are away from home.

Don't get persuaded into buying more accessories than you find absolutely necessary. Some companies have a minimum number of services you have to buy with the package. Another popular sales gimmick is to offer the cell phone at very little (or even no charge) and then lock the customer into a long-term airtime contract (e.g., up to three years). Such contracts can be difficult to terminate, unless you are willing to buy out the remaining time on your term. I briefly sold cellular phones as a job and was shocked at how many preexisting customers tried to return their phones in dismay because this clause in the sales contract had not been completely explained to them. Carefully evaluate the length of the contract term. Will a longer term remain appropriate for your needs? Instead, look into "pay as you go" plans to avoid such an obligation; here, a customer will deposit money into a plan and withdraw on this to make calls. Doing this is an ideal way to keep a better handle on your spending. On the downside, you may overlook depositing into your account and temporarily lose service, just when you may need it the most.

If you are shopping for a new or replacement phone, confirm that you will have service coverage where you will be, or plan to be physically located — if there aren't any transmission towers in your area (or in the same area you will be in if visiting your parent at a distance), a cell phone is useless. Rest assured that service is generally quite good in urban areas and it's always improving across the United States. Do note that if you are driving through the Appalachian Mountains, Adirondack Mountains, or Cascade Range on caregiving business, you may be unreachable by cell. This may be fine on a temporary basis, but make sure that you will be in a strong service area the majority of the time before purchasing a cell phone.

Another issue to look into is "roaming charges." You can be charged extra for long-distance calls made both to and from your mobile telephone, when you are outside of your primary coverage area.

Keep your conversations on your mobile phone short. While you may be tempted to chat at greater detail about matters-at-hand, or a caller may wish to monopolize your time, remember that you are paying for the convenience of the service. The extra minutes can add up quickly. Mobile phones are not designed for private conversations; for example, if you've ridden in an elevator with or sat beside someone in a restaurant who is talking on his or her cell phone, you'll know how uncomfortable this can be. Therefore, if you take a call pertaining to confidential matters, there is nothing wrong with asking your caller to hold for a minute or two until you find a quieter corner to talk. Alternatively, you can explain that you cannot talk right now but you will phone back. Be polite but firm with callers; just because they have reached you on your cell phone and you have answered the call, it does not mean that you are necessarily able to chat freely or at great length. When it comes to sharing your cell phone number, you may want to share it only with your caregiving contacts. This way, you will know that when the phone rings, you will be on-duty.

One caregiver I know also found an innovative use for her cell phone's voicemail. When her husband became ill and she visited him more often, she would often record a regular voicemail update as to her husband's condition. This way, callers could learn of his medical status without demanding too much of her time.

Keep your home landline phone, by all means, but investigate long-distance calling plans with your own telephone company. My older sister was lucky enough to find a package offering unlimited calling for a monthly flat rate and we made very good use of this. Don't wait for your telephone company to advertise a cost-effective bundle. Instead, call the company yourself and inquire about cost-saving measures.

You may want to consider booking a conference call involving a handful of people in a caregiving conversation. An advantage is that all persons involved do not have to be in the same room. If this is impossible, gather the caregivers together with numerous phone jacks. My older sister has three telephones in her home; this arrangement worked well for the family when all of us were required to either talk with each other or somebody else on our caregiving team (one of us could dial and the others could listen and join in the discussion). If you have cordless telephones, you can sit closer to each other and converse more effectively.

An alternative to conference calls is to use a speakerphone. You can collect your local circle of caregivers in one room and still involve someone far away. To remain effective, participants should be encouraged to take turns speaking. We've all been in busy rooms with several conversations going on simultaneously; it is very easy to lose track of what is being said.

By using a speakerphone, several people chiming in on a conversation can easily create chaos. True, emotions can run high during such conversations and participants can forget and just "jump in" to the discussion. Should you be recording these discussions, you'll also want to recommend that everybody present be very cognizant of not speaking when someone else is. You may want to appoint a moderator to help maintain control. Another idea would be to ask everyone in the room to raise their hands when they wish to say something. For the best sound quality when recording, try to choose a distraction-free room that has a low ceiling. Close the door to reduce outside noise or any pets or children wandering in at inopportune moments. Encourage each participant to turn off their own cell phone (or put it on "vibrate") so as not to interrupt the proceedings.

If someone cannot attend, you could also record these conversations and send the person a copy of the recording. By using a digital recorder, sessions can be recorded, uploaded to a computer, and then emailed as an audio file.

To take this idea one step further, you could even record regular caregiving updates (involving general, less time-sensitive information) and send these electronically to other family members who couldn't attend the meetings. Obviously, this will save on long-distance phone bills; the recipient will receive these immediately and can also listen at his or her convenience and replay the recording to clarify any missed information. You may want to keep these recordings for future use; for example, maybe your family wants to capture your parent's story for future generations, or in the unfortunate event of a conflict, a record can prove immeasurably useful.

Granted, having a tape recorder running during a conversation can make someone nervous. In this case, try appointing a group member to be a note-taker. These group notes can be summarized and shared with others online. From personal experience, I can recommend the Caring Bridge website (www.caringbridge.org), which I accessed when my aunt was in palliative care in California. The many miles between us made it impossible for me to visit her before she passed away; however, the regular updates (provided by other family members geographically closer to her) shared vital information and provided me some comfort with knowing what was going on with her and my relatives.

1.2 Frequent travel

Frequent traveling to visit a loved one can prove to be costly. Unlike booking a flight for a holiday, depending on your parent's situation, you won't necessarily have the luxury of pre-shopping months in advance for the least expensive airfare. Much like my younger sister did when Mom fell ill, you may have to travel at a moment's notice when an emergency strikes. With flying, costs typically rise closer to the weekend and nearing holidays (e.g., Thanksgiving and Christmas as "peak" flying times). Even the price of gas increases just before a long weekend in anticipation of people traveling out of town.

One creative way to save money on flights is to cash in your collected "frequent flyer" miles, which are often offered as incentives with various credit cards. The cardholder is awarded points, proportionate to purchases, which can be cashed in on air travel costs. Such frequent flyer points can add up quickly, can often be redeemed quite simply, and may even be transferrable (therefore, you may be able to "gift" your points to another family member to use instead).

Furthermore, traveling to a distant city or town will take time away from your own family and/or work (the latter can affect your income). For my sisters and I, flying to tend to caregiving responsibilities took only a couple of hours, but this can stretch much further. A colleague of mine previously drove between five and six hours (one way) each Friday to spend time with her aging father over the weekend. Ask yourself if you will always have that kind of time available and what type of condition your vehicle is in, such as is it comfortable for longer drives and capable of making such trips?

Boarding a Greyhound bus or riding Amtrak are other viable means of transportation. While you will be more restricted by a carrier's schedule, you can still travel between points and save on your vehicle expenses (as well as make the trip more comfortable and less physically exhausting for you).

If you live closer to your parents, you can always drive; however, you will need to consider the fuel costs and the wear-and-tear on both you and your vehicle. Driving long distances can prove to be physically and mentally taxing. Should you be driving long distances on lonely highways, remember to top up your gas tank before leaving home and keep your fully charged cell phone in your glove compartment in case of emergencies.

Depending on where you live in the United States, American winters can be harsh. If you are driving, pack a few extra layers of clothing, a shovel, a blanket or sleeping bag, candles, and matches. No matter what the season, don't forget some extra provisions to eat and drink.

Check all of your tires (including your spare) to ensure they are properly inflated. Understand how to use your vehicle's jack. With long-distance driving, ensure that your vehicle is regularly serviced and leave a planned itinerary (along with an intended route of travel) with someone back home. If you are unfamiliar with the route, don't guess. Map it before you go or use a GPS system to direct you.

If you travel to visit your parent, you will be kept busy. This, by no means, will be a vacation. If you do not have your own vehicle, rent one for your trip (or to use when you arrive). Weigh the alternatives carefully; for example, if you have a great deal of running around to do, a compact car will be less expensive on gas costs; however, a larger car will be more comfortable for your parent if he or she is riding with you. Consider the practicality of the vehicle. A van (even a minivan) will be higher off the ground and therefore may be more challenging for a senior to climb into. A four-door model will be more spacious, a larger trunk (or station wagon) can better hold a folded wheelchair, and a fold-down backseat in a hatchback can provide additional luggage space.

You may want to incorporate some fun into your rental vehicle. On one trip, I rented a vintage Volkswagen Beetle. Mom, having driven one of those in years past, was quite tickled to be shuttled around in the "bug" and to relive her memories.

If possible, sign for a rental plan where you will not be charged per mile. Some companies offer unlimited miles so shop around. Note that the extra insurance costs for a vehicle may not be necessary. Check with your own insurance agent back home to see if your coverage will also include a second car. Major credit card companies can offer additional insurance to card holders; this can be well worth looking into.

1.3 Traveling without your parent

Many family caregivers mistakenly believe they are unable to travel while caring for a loved one. Common responses include guilt of leaving a loved one and admitting that the job has become overwhelming;

and uncertainty of finding someone who can take equally good care of an aging parent. Caregivers desperately need some time away — even if only for a weekend. Granted, packing a suitcase may not be quite as easily accomplished as before you became a caregiver, but there are things you can still do to provide good, quality care.

You can arrange for home care. Begin by evaluating both professional and private home care for your parents. While many more "senior service" companies are operating now, many of these cannot guarantee providing the same employee every time (a regular visitor can become a familiar face for a senior, increase trust, and build a better relationship). Even when away from home, family caregivers can call a number of home-care companies and research them online to find out about their credentials and what kind of help they supply. Make sure to ask about a "Plan B" such as what will the company do as a contingency plan if the initially scheduled worker calls in sick or is unavailable.

You can hire a private caregiver by placing an ad in a local newspaper and asking for résumés via email. If you are not available to handle the interview, ask a sibling or someone you trust to do the interviews and check references; you can still provide your thoughts and input on each applicant from what you read in the résumés. Family caregivers hiring privately will become the employer responsible for issuing paychecks, withholding taxes, and keeping employment records. The benefit of hiring private home-care workers, besides their professional abilities to help your parent, is that they can provide you with the time and peace of mind to take some personal respite away to unwind and recharge.

While you are away, you can still offer support such as making necessary phone calls. For example, your parent may have an increasing number of medical, financial, and legal appointments. Using a cell phone, traveling caregivers can make necessary calls to book those appointments. Keep a list of key contacts (e.g., doctor, banker, long-term care home nurse) handy and share your own cell phone number in case of an emergency.

You can discuss the issues ahead of time and keep in touch with siblings who are left at home as the primary caregivers. Before leaving, have an open conversation with your family about this matter. Will they be okay with handling the increased work or will they become resentful? Get on the same page with what each family member will and can do. While traveling caregivers will be unable to provide physical help for aging adults, they can still provide vital mental and emotional help for family members. Schedule regular phone calls (or Skype meetings) to discuss matters concerning your parent. On this same topic, share your traveling schedule with other family members such as your destination, the route you will be driving, when you will arrive and depart, and where you will be staying (including a hotel/motel's phone number and room number if known). Also, consider how quickly you can return from your trip, if there is an emergency.

Contact your parent's long-term care center and tell them the dates you will be gone. If you don't already know the name of your key contact at the facility and his or her working schedule, find out so you know who to contact. Plan regular calls to ask questions and get medical updates on your parent. You will likely receive more detailed information from someone expecting your call rather than if you phone without notice. List your questions so you won't overlook asking anything and take notes. Avoid calling a long-term care center around resident mealtimes as these can be hectic times for all staff at such facilities.

1.4 Traveling with your parent

Should you and your parent travel together, inquire about companion fares. Frequently, transportation carriers offer a discounted rate on a second seat to someone accompanying a senior. If you are successful negotiating a less expensive fare, know that other senior-friendly services may be offered. Golf carts at airports can provide a lift to a senior too tired or weak to walk from one gate to another. Airlines will often allow those requiring assistance to board the airplane first. Airlines may also loan you a narrowed wheelchair, which allows for better maneuverability inside the plane.

Family caregivers can also combine transportation to ease travel stress. I remember a family trip to Mount Rainier, one of my mother's most-admired mountain peaks. With Mom's Leukemia and Dad's Alzheimer's disease, coordinating this trip took some careful and creative planning. As an answer, my two sisters, along with my niece and nephew, drove the entire distance while I flew halfway with Mom and Dad and then rented a car to drive the rest of the trip. We knew that both Mom and Dad would not be comfortable making the long road trip, especially with two raucous kids in the car, so the combination of flying and driving worked well for our situation.

We also had the luxury of having two vehicles, rather than just one, when we arrived at Mount Rainier. As the trip required a great deal of walking and Mom couldn't be on her feet a great deal, we rented a wheelchair from the Red Cross office to take with us for her use.

Before you and your loved one fly together, confirm with your doctor that it is safe to do so. High altitudes can hinder breathing. Your parent must be medically cleared. Will any medications need to be taken during the flight? If so, can you bring said medications on-board with you? What about additional health-care apparatuses? An oxygen tank, for example, may be available in a reduced size for ease of transport. If you are unsure on these matters, don't assume that everything will be fine. Call ahead to your airline or discuss it with your travel agent. Spell out the situation exactly and confirm what the exact rules are for flying. What medications and medical appara-tuses can be brought on-board? Should you have to fly repeatedly on caregiving business, double-check with each airline that these same rules apply with each trip you take.

Another thing to consider is whether your parent can last the en-tire flight without going to the bathroom. Ushering an unsteady senior from his or her seat to the rear or front of the plane to squeeze into a closet-sized facility is anything but ideal. You should consider how much movement will be required. Seat your loved one next to the aisle rather than by the window. As with medications and medical appara-tuses, you can talk to the airline company or the travel agent. Instead of reserving a seat somewhere in the middle of the plane (a tactic I will often employ to guarantee the most leg-room), perhaps it is possible to book a seat closer to the washroom to alleviate any of your parent's discomfort? Reducing a parent's liquid intake prior to take-off can reduce the number of required bathroom trips while in the air. The problem here, however, is that flying (along with certain medications that elderly people may take) can result in uncomfortable and risky dehydration. Therefore, drinking water before, during, and after a flight is encouraged; other beverages, such as caffeine, can cause a person to use the bathroom more than necessary.

While little can be done to improve a passenger's comfort in tight quarters, you can pack along a neck pillow and an extra blanket in a carry-on bag. Even a tightly rolled towel or jacket, tucked in between a person's back and the seat, can provide necessary stability and cush-ioning. Both you and your loved one will be far more comfortable on the trip if you dress in loose fitting clothes. In case of any emergencies, you may want to pack along an extra change of clothes for your parent. For longer flights where a meal may be served, confirm ahead with the airline that any parental dietary restrictions will be addressed and menu options will be available.

Another prerequisite for traveling with seniors is a checklist. Without wanting to sound harsh, don't rely on aging memories to try and remember all of the necessary details. Create a to-do list and check it to confirm everything is taken care of. Double-check the contents of your parent's suitcase or, better yet, pack it yourself to make sure that nothing is left behind.

At times like these, you cannot always trust your own memory either. As a caregiver, you will often have a great number of facts and additional information to remember. Due to these often stressful circumstances, you may not remember flight times, airline numbers, or your own suitcase. Having a checklist yourself can help you stay organized and reduce your stress.

In addition to packing your suitcases for the trip, remember to pack along plenty of patience. With slower-moving seniors, you must allow for ample time to leave home, at stopover points, and at your final destination. Confirm prior to arriving at transfer points that you will have enough time. Are your arrival and departure gates on completely opposite sides of the airport terminal? While you may be able to sprint to catch the next flight, a senior will not be able to keep up with you. Can assistance be provided to seniors to reduce the need to walk? You may be able to borrow a wheelchair. Some airports have moving sidewalks to alleviate the need for additional walking. If you are driving with your parent, you may want to map out regular rest stops to get out of the car, walk around, stretch, and go to the bathroom.

1.5 Finding accommodations

Guest accommodation for visiting caregivers must also be addressed. Where will you stay when you arrive? Newer seniors' apartments may feature furnished guest suites — a very clever idea for visiting family members staying on a temporary basis. Considering the alternative of booking a few nights in a local hotel, the option of a guest suite is far more cost-effective, comfortable, and convenient. Because of those very same reasons, however, these guest suites may be reserved by others. Remember that long weekends and holidays may bring more visiting caregivers, so demand for the guest suites can increase. You'll need to book the suite as early as possible to avoid disappointment.

When staying in a seniors' home guest suite, a visiting caregiver can also scope out the building and witness the staff at work at different times of the day. This can provide you more peace of mind. If space permits, you could always "camp out" with your parents. My parent's home fortunately had a spare room. Without an extra bed, or even a couch or a futon, a visiting caregiver would be relegated to a sleeping bag with a couch pillow on the floor. For the convenience and comfort of visiting family caregivers, you could store an inflatable mattress, an extra pillow, and a few blankets in a closet.

If you do prefer a real bed, locate a hotel or motel located nearby. As with airline flights, know that your credit card's frequent flyer points will often cover a percentage of your accommodation costs. If you are working with a travel agent, inquire about package deals in which you can book a flight, a hotel room, and a rental car for a better rate. Numerous travel websites exist as well, so shop around at sites such as Expedia, Travelocity, Kayak, and Trivago. If you stay over a weekend, will your travel price increase or be reduced? While credit card reward points typically cannot be used over holidays (airlines prefer to save plane seats for paying passengers), there are ample opportunities to take advantage of this offer throughout the rest of the year.

Should you expect to be visiting your parent often and staying at the same hotel repeatedly, introduce yourself to the hotel manager and explain that you will be a regular guest. As such, you may be able to negotiate a better price for a few nights' stay or perhaps upgrade to a larger room. It never hurts to ask about an offered discount either. Many times, hotels will offer you a better rate if they are not booked solid. For the hotel manager, getting even partial payment for a room is better than having that room sit empty.

2. What to Do When You Get There

After arriving, ensure that you meet with your parent's neighbors and friends. Exchange phone numbers and email addresses with them because these individuals can provide a much-needed set of helpful eyes and ears after you leave. Consider providing your parent's trusted neighbors with an extra set of house keys to use in case of any urgent situation. Other people you will want to introduce yourself to include your parent's mail carrier and barber or hairstylist. The mail carrier may be able to alert you if your parent's mailbox has not been emptied for a few days; the barber or hairstylist can let you know if Mom or Dad doesn't show up for a regular appointment.

Attend as many area functions with your parent as possible during your visit. This will get your parent out and active within the local community. Help your parent join a seniors' center, which can offer friendships and activities. Suggest classes or workshops that your parent may be interested in taking; instructors may be willing to welcome your parent in to simply audit a class for no credit. Investigate local volunteering opportunities where your parent could share his or her experience with others.

My mother and father got involved with Meals on Wheels. This is a program that prepares and provides meals to housebound seniors. While Mom and Dad remained as capable cooks themselves, they volunteered as drivers which worked out very well for a good number of reasons — doing this involved them in the community, it kept them both active, it allowed them to meet and socialize with others, and it provided a chance to better learn their way around their new city. What volunteer opportunities exist for your parents?

If your parent has religious beliefs, attend church services with him or her. You could ask among the congregation (or advertise in the church newsletter) for a friendly home visitor. Can someone from the church call or visit every few days to check in on your parents?

Look into local service providers such as a regular housekeeper to come in to clean, launder clothes, and perform other light household duties. This can be of immense help (aging bodies don't bend over so well to plug a vacuum cleaner in or are less able to carry a heavy laundry basket), not to mention the person can provide some welcome company for your parents. That same housekeeper may also be called on to cook meals if that is a service he or she provides. Hired housekeeping help may also support visiting caregivers by running outside errands for them.

You may also want to consider hiring someone or finding a volunteer that will mow your parent's lawn or shovel snow. Not only does this reduce the heavier work for your mother or father, it reduces the risk of injuries incurred. For example, your parent may easily slip and fall on a snow-covered sidewalk while trying to clear away ice and snow. Lifting snow can also cause back strain. If your hired hand has his or her own lawn mower, rake, and snow shovel for use, all the better. Having such tools around may tempt your parent to tackle the work.

Securing a home-care service to provide regular help with dressing or bathing your parent may also be something you need to consider. More seniors' services are being offered on a mobile basis; I have personally seen professionals who go to a seniors' homes to provide haircutting, glasses repair, dentistry, and pedicures. Check your phone book, see who is advertising in your local seniors' newspaper, make some calls, and inquire into the availability and pricing of such services.

3. Find the Necessary Information and Documents

Meet all the professionals currently involved with your parent's care; these may include a doctor, lawyer, and banker or financial planner. During my visits to see my parents, I always packed along a notebook and a couple of pens — having more than one pen meant I would always have an extra, should the other one run out at an inopportune moment. When I met with the banker, financial planner, doctor, and realtor, I always made copious notes about our conversation. In addition, I found the notebook handy to record thoughts, observances (e.g., Mom was more tired today than yesterday and Dad had remembered what day of the week it was), and questions I should ask. When it comes to asking questions, don't be shy! Keep asking until you completely understand the answers. Advocate and clarify; you are doing this on your loved one's behalf. Professionals of all types often speak in industry jargon which, unless you have gained related knowledge, you often cannot comprehend.

When talking to the banker, collect necessary banking information such as the bank location, account numbers, and the value of additional investment holdings. Don't overlook any credit cards and foreign accounts.

Confirm the whereabouts of all necessary documents such as your parent's will(s), birth certificate, and Social Security card and ensure these are kept secure. A common storage area for these documents is a bank safety deposit box, so make sure you obtain an extra key to take back home with you. If there is no bank safety deposit box, purchase a small, fireproof safe for home storage. As an extra precaution, photocopy or scan all these documents you find and keep these copies at a separate, safe location; you never know when you might need them. (See Chapter 5 for more information about locating important documents.)

4. Check the Safety of Your Parent's Home

When you are visiting, remain alert to the safety issues in your parent's home — both the interior and the exterior. For example, frayed or loose carpeting can be a dangerous tripping hazard; extra furniture may only occupy space and not serve any useful purpose.

Observe your parent getting in and out of his or her chair; if extensive effort is required, maybe it is time to replace it. Cushy couch cushions can prove to be very comfortable, but they can actually trap a senior who is too weak to stand. While it can be difficult to dismiss any sentimental attachments you may have to an old couch or rocking chair, do so. If you, or another family member, choose not to adopt your parent's furniture, it is far better to sell or donate tables, chairs, and shelves rather than place them in storage indefinitely. The monthly fee for secured lock-up can add up quickly. Save yourself the money and call on local nonprofit associations; they may be able to suggest or find a good home for your parent's old armchair. Better yet, maybe they will even arrange pick up.

Check for any lightbulbs that need to be replaced. You may find that you need to install a new lighting fixture to remove dangerous shadows in the hallway — aging eyes aren't as sharp as they once were. Do you need to remove a mirror at the end of the hall? A somewhat cognitively impaired senior may mistake his or her reflection in the mirror as another person walking towards them and become startled, alarmed, or frightened. For that same reason, a bathroom mirror may also need to be removed.

Check for leaks in the roof or around windows or doors. Replace broken windows, which can allow for cold air to enter the home. Walk through and around your parent's home (and then do so a second time); verify the smoke alarm is working properly.

No senior's home inspection would be complete without visiting the bathroom. With wet floors, this room can become dangerous. Install grab bars around the shower and bathtub. Towel racks screwed into walls may seem secure; however, they can be easily torn loose. Even shower curtains can be grabbed by a bathing senior to save himself or herself from falling. Place a nonskid mat in the shower and tub. Replace flooring, if necessary, and avoid slippery tiles. Replace an aging bathtub with a walk-in tub instead where the senior can step in, close the door, and enjoy a good soak. A Jacuzzi bathtub's hot water jets can be very therapeutic for sore joints and nagging injuries.

Are there stairs inside or outside the home? Explore the possibility of installing a mechanical stair lift, which can smoothly carry your loved one up or down a flight of stairs. Alternatively, consider if a wheelchair ramp can be placed at the front, side, or rear of the home. If land space is limited, know that a wheelchair ramp does not have to extend straight out; it can be built to double back on itself or even curl around. Ensure that the incline is not too steep and that the ramp features secure handrails, so that your parents can pull themselves up, if need be.

Homes should not only be comfortable for the residents, they must also be safe. If your parents remain living at home, be fully prepared to make any adaptations necessary for their safety. While you may hesitate to pay for home reconstruction, do know that many of these necessary changes will increase the property's value. Look for a qualified contractor, ask for and check references, and get written estimates prior to any work being started. A Self-Counsel book, *Aging Safely in Your Home*, has more information on this. An often-overlooked source of financial help can be local governments that may have rebate programs and grants for helping seniors stay in their own homes longer and safely.

Worksheet 3: Home Safety Checklist will help you make sure that your loved one is safe and has ease of mobility in his or her own home.

5. Respect the Decision That Not Everyone Wants to Relocate

I was lucky that when my parent's medical situations arose, my mother and father understood the need to return to their former city although it was not their dream retirement destination. They realized and accepted how their three children could provide much better care from nearby rather than from afar. Should your parents remain obstinate, please take a page out of my family's caregiving manual and

Worksheet 3
Home Safety Checklist

If your parent is not fully ready for institutionalized care, one option may be for her or him to remain at home. For your loved one's safety, comfort, and ease of mobility around the home, you will have to realistically evaluate the home then make some adjustments. In addition to evaluating the home in question, you may also need to carefully assess your parent's abilities to remain independent at home. In no specific order, here are a few recommendations:

- ❏ Place nonskid mats inside and outside of a shower or bathtub.
- ❏ Mount grab bars on the walls around the shower, bathtub, and toilet.
- ❏ Install a smoke alarm (closer to the bedroom is preferable); check and replace the battery regularly.
- ❏ Purchase a home fire extinguisher. Keep this in a central, easily accessible spot (e.g., your parent's kitchen) and check this regularly to ensure proper operation.
- ❏ Remove throw rugs from the floor.
- ❏ Secure or remove loose carpeting.
- ❏ Replace patterned carpeting (which may be confusing to older eyes).
- ❏ Provide extra phones (e.g., having one phone in the kitchen and another in the bedroom gives a senior more accessible choices when needed).
- ❏ De-clutter the surroundings. Remove unneeded furniture and create an open path for walking or wheelchair/walker use.
- ❏ Replace water faucet taps with handle levers for ease of operation.
- ❏ Move dishes and glasses to lower shelves to reduce unnecessary reaching.
- ❏ Replace dishes and glasses with plastic products to reduce accidental breakage.
- ❏ Consider installing a stair lift to ease access to upper and lower floors.
- ❏ Paint the tops of stairs a lighter color (or choose a brighter tone of carpeting) to provide better visibility.
- ❏ Secure/tighten all staircase handrails.
- ❏ Place a list of family and emergency phone numbers conspicuously by the telephone or attach it to your parent's refrigerator door as many emergency responders will check there first.

❏ Replace a full-sized vacuum cleaner with a built-in system (to reduce the need to lug a heavy machine around the house).

❏ Clean the refrigerator and/or pantry on a regular basis. Dispose of spoiled food (note that even canned foods have a "best before" date for safe consumption).

❏ Install a wheelchair ramp, if necessary, outside the house.

❏ Transfer cereals or grains from boxes to sealed plastic containers for safer storage.

❏ Tuck any extension cords safely behind furniture rather than stretch them across an open floor. This will reduce the risk of tripping.

❏ Hire a reputable housekeeper to assist with cleaning.

◇◇◇

share the workload with other relatives, if possible. In my case, my sisters and I rotated as full-time caregiver for Mom and Dad prior to their move.

This idea, resulting in each of us taking a temporary leave from work to focus on our parent's needs, resulted from ongoing discussion. Part of each relocated sibling's responsibility as temporary full-time caregiver included a regular phone call to report back to the family. When I was working in this role, I would often take a few minutes and review my notes from the day to better prepare. We made excellent use of my older sister's flat-rate long-distance calling plan during that time — the family member visiting could call at an appointed time and my sister would then call back (thus saving on the long-distance calling charges).

Granted, your parents may not be as obliging as mine were. If your mother or father does not wish to move, there is little you can do about it. In this case, the need for long-distance caregiving practices and open lines of communication become even more necessary. Hiring a part-time or full-time local caregiver to help can be a very viable solution. One job requirement for a distant caregiver could be to participate in a weekly conference call to you and your siblings to share any news or concerns.

If, however, your parent's or your own finances are limited, you may not be able to hire private care. You may also feel that caring for your own parents remains your own obligation. In this case, can you relocate yourself, even temporarily, to help tend to parental needs? Openly discuss your need for a leave of absence with your employer. You may be able to negotiate a discount with a local hotel if you wish to stay long-term; however, you may be more comfortable renting an apartment for three to six months, or more if necessary. For furnishings, you can rent furniture — items can be delivered, and picked up when you no longer require them. You may also have the option of renting a furnished apartment.

Aging parents are not the only ones who move away. Adult children can relocate as well. This may be done for any number of reasons such as a job offer, a blossoming relationship, educational training, or simply due to personal preference. If it's a sibling or other caregiver in your circle, respect the person's choice to move away. While you can reasonably request a person's involvement with caregiving responsibilities, you must also respect his or her choice to remain distant.

6. Emotional Distance

In addition to physical distance, caregivers can experience emotional distance. For any number of personal reasons, family members may feel uncomfortable stepping into a caregiver's shoes. In such cases, do not force anyone to take on a caregiving job unwillingly. A reluctant caregiver is a resistant caregiver, which is not helpful. Caregiving requires ability, trust, desire, and dedication so if a sibling does not want to help, it's best to accept this and carry on.

Arguing is often pointless and may only drive a dagger deeper into teetering family relationships. Instead, talk openly with the other person, understand his or her reasons for the decision, and be accepting. Often, these reasons will be quite sound. Try compromising to avoid family hostility. It's better to accept the familial differences now than to face possible alienation later.

When working closely with other family members, expect to encounter opposition. You are all at very close quarters at these times and not everybody may agree that one approach is the best direction to take. Consensus may be more difficult to reach than you might imagine. Families can and will argue. There were heated conversations that occurred between my sisters and I; however, we eventually decided to accept other points of view, negotiate, and compromise.

Arguing might occur within your own family, but you must remember that caregiving is not all about you; instead, it is about your loved one. Know that you do not have to win all the arguments, suggest the right option, or be right absolutely every time. As human beings, we don't like to admit our own mistakes and how we might be wrong, but park your own pride and ask yourself the following questions before you get mad:

- How will your parent best benefit?
- What is most important to your parent?
- What values does your parent hold dear?
- What would your parent do in a similar situation?

Considering what your parent would do in a similar situation helps to put you in his or her perspective. In making the same choice as your parent would, it may help to put your parent more at ease. With caregiving, one of the last things you want is your parent or siblings to feel threatened or become defensive. This will make caregiving even more challenging. Thinking in parental terms may make difficult family decisions easier and can often be more beneficial in the long term.

On the subject of distance caregiving, pay attention to distant siblings who may drop in irregularly and come brimming with ideas and recommendations. While you may admire this enthusiasm, take note that this person is often not the senior's primary caregiver who is local and steers the ship on a far more regular basis. Someone dropping in and, essentially, taking over may be viewed as someone stepping on the primary caregiver's toes. Even the most well-meaning advice and efforts from a distant caregiver can be taken the wrong way and the primary caregiver may take offense. You don't need any additional hostility at these times.

Distant caregivers, therefore, should remember that their role may be support to the primary caregiver. While they may be handed the wheel of the ship, a better role for them is that of second officer. To avoid a small skirmish or outright war between a distant and primary caregiver, try talking about things before a visit. Brainstorming ideas on how best to manage one's time during a brief visit is a good idea, but it is equally, or more important to lay out expectations of the visiting caregiver before he or she comes to call.

By having a to-do list ahead of time, a visiting caregiver can focus on and complete certain jobs and feel that his or her time has been well-spent (everyone likes to be appreciated). If all the distance caregiver and primary caregiver do is squabble for the first couple of days of a four- or five-day visit, this will be wasted time and all parties involved will become more frustrated. Instead, use this time more productively to focus on the health and/or lifestyle choices for your aging parent.

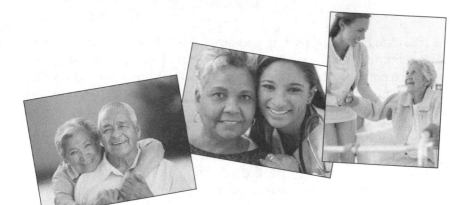

Chapter 3
Finding Suitable Accommodations

"Home is a shelter from storms — all sorts of storms."

– William J. Bennett

The move is imminent. Your parent has weakened, become sick, or has outgrown services provided at home. Where your parent goes depends on his or her current and future needs. Different levels of care exist, so you must ensure that you make the proper choice — the chosen facility must be suitable for both the immediate and forthcoming situations.

Know that this time can be immensely trying for caregivers. When I helped move my father into long-term care (a locked Alzheimer's unit and his final home), the stark reality hit me hard that he was not going to get any better.

As a senior grows older, he or she may need additional help with physical and medical issues, which care-home employees are qualified to do rather than untrained family members. Realistically, moving a senior into a care home may prove to be best for him or her and the family caregivers. A senior's current home may be too large to take care of, so downsizing and moving will be necessary. Looking after a home, especially one that is also aging, can prove to become expensive with increased maintenance costs. While your parent may fight to stay in his or her own home, any required retrofits to the home to become more senior friendly can also break the bank.

Remembering my own parents' situation, they both stubbornly fought against losing their independence. Thinking back, I realize that some of their resistance was simply due to not wanting to give up their warm and scenic island retirement home. I suspect that they may also have felt resentment from not being able to function self-sufficiently, confusion (especially on my father's part as he did not completely grasp that Mom was sick), embarrassment from needing help from their children, and fear of the future. While adult children often believe that their parents are simply being "difficult" or obstinate at such times, these feelings are perfectly natural and can be effectively addressed to help with a smoother transition.

Communication at this time is critical. Listen to any concerns raised and choose your own words carefully. For instance, my sisters and I approached our parents as a unified group and explained we were concerned about their health and we could provide far better care and support for them if they lived closer to us.

Don't stop with just communicating with your aging parents; talk with your siblings as well to understand where they are at — due to their own family matters, work situations, and geographical location, they may be unable to drop everything at a moment's notice to help pack and move your parent.

1. The Different Types of Living Arrangements

No matter where you live in the United States, and whether you are new to caregiving or well-established in this role, you will hear various terms for seniors' living choices. Where do you begin?

With many diverse care options available, it is easy enough for a caregiver to be confused as to where to place an aging mother or father to receive the best care. To make matters worse, there can be a great deal of crossover in services provided between care facilities. How do you know which facility will provide the best care for your parent? How much care will be provided in the future? These questions can be difficult to answer as nothing is certain. By thoroughly researching the specific health condition, you can have a better idea of what can be expected. For further clarification, I will explain several key terms you will likely hear as your parent's condition progresses.

1.1 Aging in place

The senior will remain living in his or her home for as long as possible. There are advantages to aging in place such as the familiarity and comfort of staying in one's home, but this type of situation should be monitored closely.

Certain rooms, or even second floors or basements, may become completely inaccessible and even standard doorways (especially in older homes) may be too narrow to allow for a wheelchair or a walker to pass through. Light switches, counters, and cupboards may be too high for a senior in a wheelchair to reach. Homes can be modified to allow seniors to stay in them for longer, but doing this can take time and become very expensive. These drawbacks could be outweighed by the fact that the senior will know the neighbors and likely have a good network of contacts. With a few modifications (e.g., a wheelchair ramp or emergency-response system being installed), a senior can remain living at home safely.

1.2 Elder villages

For seniors (aged 55 and older) living at home who may be unable to complete certain tasks, the village option is now available. Seniors remain in their own homes and pay an annual fee. In return, the seniors can have access to a bank of volunteers who can lend a hand with any number of odd jobs including providing transportation, completing light home repairs, shoveling snow, and picking up groceries. Seniors requiring more extensive help are not ignored or forgotten; they can be referred to outside service providers (who may discount their rates for those living in an elder village).

America's first senior's village was established in Boston in 2001. Today, more than 56 villages exist in the United States, with even more in development.[1]

1.3 Naturally occurring retirement communities

Naturally occurring retirement communities do not start out as senior communities, but become them. This occurs as the residents remain at home and continue to age. Programs and services (financially

---

1 "Villages: Helping People Age in Place," Martha Thomas, *AARP The Magazine*, accessed April 2015.
   http://www.aarp.org/home-garden/livable-communities/info-04-2011/villages-real-social-network.html

supported by private and public funding sources) can be similar to those offered in elder villages; however, will be introduced over the course of time and can vary from one naturally occurring retirement community to the next (as they are specific to residents).

1.4 Independent living

As the name "independent living" implies, residents in this type of facility remain physically and mentally able to manage their own needs. Commonly, the seniors' independent living facility is either an apartment or condominium complex in which seniors are freed from doing home maintenance, mowing the lawn, shoveling snow, and so on.

1.5 Assisted living

Assisted living can prove to be ideal for seniors who will require some limited help or assistance with daily activities. With assisted living, a senior can receive more hands-on health care and management. Staff in such facilities can assist with medication reminders and dressing a resident.

We chose an assisted living property for Mom and Dad as their first stop. While my parents lived in their own apartment within the building, a group dining room offered the convenience of not having to cook. They also had the camaraderie of dining with other residents. Meals were included in the monthly rent; however, there was a charge for additional meals or snacks. In addition, there was a "great room" with a pool table and big screen television, which also provided a communal setting for guest speakers and exercise classes.

1.6 Continuing care retirement communities

A senior's needs may change over the course of time and moving him or her may result in a further distance between family members. With continuing care retirement communities, senior residents can move under the same roof and receive higher levels of care, when necessary. Moving is hard for anybody — especially seniors. Moving to another room just down the hall can effectively reduce the level of stress (felt by both seniors and caregivers) as well as the associated mental and physical decline that seniors can experience following a move.

There is an initial cost for residents to buy a unit in a continuing care retirement community and further monthly fees will be added (e.g., monthly condominium fees). Collected fees will be saved and can be used towards future care needs.

1.7 Nursing homes (long-term care facilities)

Nursing homes (also known as long-term care facilities) are typically the final stop for a senior who has advanced health issues and cannot continue living independently at home. Nursing home rooms are either private or shared (private rooms are often more expensive) and the senior or family caregiver will pay a monthly fee to cover the cost of care.

Nursing homes are best suited for seniors requiring high-level care. Nursing home staff will often include licensed physicians, nurses, occupational therapists, and physical therapists.

2. Things to Consider When Searching for Accommodations for Your Parent

Finding the right accommodations for your parent may cause some confusion because there remains a great deal of crossover between each type of facility. Similar to my own situation, you may be required to move your parent more than once. Moving a senior can often be quite challenging; you might doubt that you are making the best decision, and you might face resistance from your parent who may fear what lies ahead.

Looking at long-term care options is daunting for caregivers. I almost envied my father, who was not even aware of the forthcoming moves and the amount of work involved to relocate him. As a caregiver, you should not jump into a decision too hastily because with poor judgment, both you and your parent can be negatively affected. You've likely heard the expression, "When you fail to plan, you plan to fail." This is very true. By failing to plan properly, your parent could be receiving inadequate care, paying excessive care costs, or living in a less-than-ideal facility.

I learned that the best route to take was to tour the facilities of choice and ask specific questions. When I was exploring available facilities for Dad, I discovered that many of the properties only offered group tours once or twice per week. If you have ever taken a group tour while on vacation, you'll know that you are often rushed through, which doesn't allow you to take time to view or sufficiently explore the attraction or historic site. Push for an independent tour. While group tours may be more convenient for care-center staff, the times and dates may not be convenient for you and you do not have to be totally obliging. When being hustled through a property, you may not have a chance to ask all of your questions. Although you may feel uncomfortable raising certain questions, you have every right to ask and find out the answers before you make any decision.

Don't just settle for the mapped-out tour where you will only see what is shown. Investigate less-populated areas including stairwells and closets; are these swept and mopped regularly? Ask to see the kitchen and food-service areas. Is this a healthy and sanitary environment? Are the public washrooms cleaned? Tour a property with all your senses — what do you see, smell, and hear?

Don't overlook how accommodating the facility will be to your parent's lifestyle. Does your parent have any idiosyncrasies that may require addressing? As an example, both my parents enjoyed sipping a glass of wine with their dinner — a harmless matter — yet, we had to pass on several independent living properties with communal resident dining where management was not comfortable with any public alcohol consumption.

To better prepare yourself for the choice ahead, you will want to speak with other family members of the residents. As a casual visitor, you will face resistance from the staff if you ask for the names and phone numbers of the residents' relatives. The care-center staff must abide by the *Freedom of Information Act* and will not release any personal information.

In my opinion, there is nothing wrong with striking up a friendly conversation with residents while you are touring a property. Introduce yourself and your parent as a potential new resident and casually ask for opinions. Some of the best information available about services comes from word-of-mouth from someone already using that same service. When it comes to choosing a long-term care facility for your parent, you can never ask too many questions. Remember, there are no foolish questions and, chances are, that one question will naturally lead to the next. If you do not understand an answer, or you feel that you have received an incomplete reply, press for more information.

If you have no idea of where or how to begin searching for a long-term care facility, ask for recommendations from others. Your family physician, hospital social workers, seniors' associations, and friends who are also caregivers can all be excellent sources of information.

If you are comparing different sites, take a notepad with you on each trip to record your thoughts and observations. You may also want to make a few copies of Worksheet 6: Researching Long-Term Care Facilities (see the end of section 2.11 or use the form in the download kit) so as to have something to refer to for each site tour. Keep your notes together in either a binder or file folder.

You can also carry a small, digital recorder to verbally record any comments you may have. As with note taking, you may wish to record any self-talk when you are back in your vehicle.

Should you have the choice when it comes to where to move your parent, carefully weigh the options. Yes, it is natural for a person to be attracted to the biggest and brightest facility; however, ensure that you are placing your parent in proper care, which is dependent on his or her needs. If your parent is able to tour the facilities with you and give an opinion, by all means get his or her input. However, if your parent is unable to accompany you, or share coherent thoughts, ask yourself if he or she would be pleased with the accommodations.

The information and questions in the following sections will help you and your parent decide if a care center is the right choice.

2.1 Evaluate your parent's needs, wants, and resources

By carefully considering your parent's current physical and mental capabilities, as well as what may potentially lie ahead, you are well on your way to selecting an appropriate setting for your aging mother or father. Ask your parent's doctor for a complete diagnosis and appropriate accommodation choices so that you can be best prepared. If your parent remains cognitively aware, ask him or her about living preferences and then seek options from there.

Ask yourself: Will your parent be happy living at this facility? Know that your parent may balk at even hearing the idea of moving into long-term care, but he or she may be much happier and healthier as a result.

Understand that long-term care is a business and that there are costs involved. Look at your parent's entire financial picture (e.g., accumulated savings in a bank account, investments, building and property holdings, and continued income through a pension). Consider the following questions:

- Can your parent or the family incur these costs without financial hardship?
- Are there any hidden costs (e.g., to cover a private room or additional care)?
- How likely are these costs of care to rise over the next few years and by how much?
- Can your family or parent afford all types of care in the long term?

2.2 Consider the options

By visiting each facility you are considering, you can collect a great deal of information. Take your parent with you and ask for his or her opinion; even if your parent doesn't say too much, you can always observe his or her body language visiting the long-term care home. Compare your findings carefully:

- Is the level of care appropriate?
- Does your parent like the facility?
- Where is the property located?
- What amenities are offered?
- What is the staff-to-resident ratio both during the day and overnight?
- What is the cost of care?

Negotiation on a final choice may be called for amongst you and your family. Such negotiation is most effective when your parent remains well and is more independent.

As your parent ages and declines further, he or she may require more specialized care and you may have more limited choices. For example, when I was faced with moving Dad into an Alzheimer's unit, there was little I could do. My sisters and I were resigned to taking the first bed that became available for him. There was nothing else for Dad and we couldn't simply leave him where he was.

2.3 Review the location

Location can prove to be important for both you and your parent. Before we moved Dad into continuing care, he and my mother lived at an independent living seniors' residence. While meals, laundry service, medication reminders, and more were available, residents were not required to use them.

One of the important factors of this property was the close proximity to the city's scenic river valley. When Dad was still mobile, I accompanied him on many walks along these paths. An avid and strong hiker in his younger years, Dad still kept up a great pace and obviously enjoyed stretching his legs. As things turned out, this building was located just across the river from the hospital where Mom began receiving regular blood transfusions and these same paths became a good pastime to keep Dad distracted and busy.

It is paramount to carefully evaluate the location of a building:

- Is it a suitable location for you to visit your parent?
- Will it be convenient for you to take your parent on regular outings (e.g., church services)?
- Is the property close to a hospital?
- Is the building in a safe neighborhood for older people?

Is there a passenger loading and unloading zone located in front of the property's front door? You should be able to park there temporarily when either picking up or dropping off your parent. An additional bonus would be a sheltered loading zone to protect your parent from bad weather such as rain or snow. (My parent's first home when they returned from Victoria offered a waiting zone in front of the building as well as underground parking on-site, which was very convenient for visiting caregivers.)

On the subject of property location, another question to ask yourself is whether there is ample visitor parking (e.g., reserved spaces or on a first-come, first-serve basis). What I had initially perceived to be a large parking lot at my father's facility proved to fill up quite quickly as both care staff and visiting family members parked there. If you do not drive, you will have to find out about access by public transit. What is the scheduling? When Dad was alive, I wasn't driving. My evening and weekend visits to see him required more time and planning on my part as transit service was reduced during these times.

2.4 Check the maintenance and cleanliness

When you first arrive, check the appearance and condition of the building. Ask yourself the following questions to ascertain the effectiveness and conscientiousness of the building's cleaning and maintenance staff:

- If you are visiting in the winter, are the sidewalks cleared of ice and snow and sanded?
- In summer, is the outside grass neatly trimmed?
- Are there cracks in the sidewalks?
- Could the exterior walls use a fresh coat of paint?
- Is the facility clean and well-lit?
- How thorough is the janitorial or cleaning staff?
- Are spills mopped up immediately or left ignored?
- Are there any unpleasant odors?

2.5 Observe care staff interactions with others

Observe the interaction between care staff and residents. How the staff work with and manage the current residents can demonstrate how they will work with and manage your parent. You want your loved one to be properly taken care of and to feel welcome in the facility, so ask yourself the following questions:

- As you enter the facility, do you feel welcomed?
- Is there a general office to which family members can report?
- Are you greeted immediately? (If nothing else, look for eye contact.)
- Is the staff friendly? Did at least one staffer smile and say "hello" to you?
- While the staff may not have the time to mingle with all of the residents, is there acknowledgment at some level (perhaps a warm smile, greeting, or quick adjustment of a pillow in a wheelchair)?
- Do staff call residents by their first names? (When Dad's care staff became aware of his professional teaching background, many of them liked to call him "Professor.")

- How qualified are the care staff? Remember that the number of qualified staff can be reduced in the evenings or overnight as a cost-saving measure.

- Do the residents interact well with each other?

- Are staff working with residents or chatting amongst themselves?

- What is the level of care available and the ratio of care staff to residents? (Note that the number of overnight staff may be reduced.)

- Are there any restrictions to when family members can visit?

2.6 Take note of additional services

Consider whether or not the facility has any additional services for residents within the building:

- Are there hairdressing and nail-care services on-site? When are these services available?

- Does the facility offer physiotherapy?

- Does the facility offer regular activities and/or outings for seniors and/or in-house entertainment?

- If your parent is of a religious faith, does the center cater to various denominations? If so, how? Is there a chapel on-site?

- What other activities are available and how often are they planned? Will your parent find these activities enjoyable and stimulating?

- Is there a sunroom or patio? (The balcony at my father's Alzheimer's care center was completely screened, which reduced annoying bugs.)

- Are care meetings between family and facility staff routinely scheduled? These are excellent opportunities for family caregivers to be updated on their parent's health condition as well as to ask any pressing questions.

- What is the process for family members who wish to make suggestions and/or air grievances?

- Is extended care available, if need be?

- Can a senior be transferred within the same facility to receive specialized treatment?

2.7 Look at the resident rooms

View your parent's potential room. Consider the size, shape, and location of this room within the building. Some things to evaluate when viewing the room include the following:

- Window placement and accessibility: Your parent may find an eastern exposure pleasing for the morning sunshine. Can the window be opened or is it permanently bolted shut? Depending on your parent's mental awareness, an open window could pose a risk; however, a warm summer's breeze blowing through the room or the laughter of children playing nearby can by very pleasant and therapeutic. If your parent is confined to a bed, is the window still close enough to offer a view outside?

- Can the bed be moved or adjusted for additional comfort?

- How much space is available for additional furnishings?

- Can any space-saving modifications be done inside the room? (My family was successful with having facility maintenance staff attach a couple of new shelves to the wall above Dad's bed.)

- Will this room be shared with another resident? If so, how is the room divided (e.g., an actual wall or a privacy curtain around each bed)?

- Are there any restrictive columns/pillars?

- Is the bathroom shared or independent?

- How much closet space is provided?

- Will the room temperature be either too warm or too cold for your parent? Can residents control their own personal room temperatures or is there a central control behind the main nurse's desk and inaccessible to those who don't work in the facility? It is quite possible that all residents will not agree on a temperature compromise, so having a separate thermostat in each room can be both advantageous and convenient for residents.

With my father's lifelong connection to books, my family supplied him with a small bookcase and asked the facility's maintenance staff to install some small wheels on the bottom. Even when the shelves were fully laden with books (although Dad eventually couldn't read, we felt he still recognized books and found comfort with them being there), it was easy enough to roll the bookshelf away from the wall to sweep and mop behind it.

With Dad's room, the curtains around each bed provided the only separation from his roommate. While more privacy would have been nice, it was not our biggest concern. Though your parent's comfort and preferences are important, finding the perfect set of circumstances is rare — if not impossible. Be prepared to compromise or prioritize, but if something is very important to your parent, do what you can to help accommodate his or her preference — this may change his or her experiences in a facility dramatically.

2.8 Observe mealtimes

Mealtimes at seniors' homes can be very busy, but they can also be excellent times for you to tour. Consider the following questions:

- What is offered for meals?
- How is the food served to residents?
- Is the menu varied and appealing?
- Can the facility's kitchen accommodate for any menu preferences, food allergies, or diet requirements?
- If your parent is a strict vegetarian, will the staff prepare nutritious meals and offer a variety for this type of diet?
- If your parent cannot hold cutlery tightly or chew food properly, can assistance be provided (e.g., modified cutlery or food served chopped, diced, or pureed)?
- Can you sample the food yourself?

2.9 Calculate the cost

You will need to find out what the cost is for regular care, budget for it, and then ascertain if there are any hidden costs involved. The flat fee that your parent is paying may only cover the basic necessities; typically, anything "extra" will cost extra. (See section 3. for more information about costs.)

It can also prove to be worthwhile to check if these costs can be subsidized. Remember, while you will naturally want the best care for your parent, it can be very expensive. Ongoing medical treatment may be necessary and, without insurance, you or your loved one will be left incurring much of the cost.

In my father's case, his long-term care center offered sliding scale payments based on income. Those residents who could pay more were expected to do so while others were offered a discounted monthly rate. Proof of a resident's total income had to be provided.

2.10 Consider safety

Safety is an important topic to consider when it comes to the care of your loved one. Ask the following questions:

- When was the building last inspected?
- If there is an elevator? If so, when was it last serviced?
- How often are building and elevator inspections scheduled?
- What is the emergency evacuation procedure? Although Dad and other residents were on the third floor, I was assured that they would be safely ushered down a flight of stairs, if need be. In remembering that many of the residents were confined to wheelchairs and were cognitively impaired, I now wonder just how effectively this would have been done.
- Does the center have emergency lighting in case of a power outage?
- Are resident medication and toxic cleaning supplies safely locked up and out of reach of those who may be confused?
- Is the building well-lit?
- Are there automatic sensors that trigger outside lights at night when someone is approaching?
- Is the main entry brightly lit? This can provide additional safety and security to a resident coming home in the evening.
- Is the center's front door locked? Visiting family members may need an extra key or tap in a security passcode to open the door.

2.11 Shortlist your top choices

Shortlisting your top choices can be very similar to conducting job interviews where you will personally meet with the most likely candidates, perhaps call them back for a second interview, and then hire the best person for the job. The key here is the personal contact. You can learn much more about a facility by visiting it, finding a contact there, and having a face-to-face meeting than you can by speaking to staff on the telephone. In other words, visit each potential facility so as to make the best, the most logical, and the most educated decision for your mother or father.

Worksheet 4: Researching Long-Term Care Facilities will help you make a wise choice from your options.

3. Affording the Cost of Care

You might be wondering what it costs for long-term seniors' housing. At the time of this book's publication, the ranges were the following:

- Independent living: $1,500 to $3,500 per month.

- Assisted living: $2,500 to $4,000 per month.

- Full-scale nursing/long-term care home: $4,000 to $8,000 per month.

Through inflation, these costs will not decrease. Depending on the location, the services provided, and the available amenities of such facilities as well as the future health-care needs of your parent, it is impossible to provide an exact figure, but do know that senior care can prove to be very expensive.

No matter where you place your aging parent, the associated costs of accommodation and provided care can become expensive. Long-term care is a pricey proposition. If your parent has accumulated sufficient savings during his or her life, you can draw from these funds as needed; however, that well may run dry sooner than you might expect. Consider the following recommendations to save some money.

3.1 Explore sliding scale care costs

Does your facility of choice charge a flat fee per month or does the cost vary based on a senior's income? With Dad's final home, the residents' family members were required to share their parent's income and the monthly rent was then assessed. Unfortunately, Dad's income (including his pension) was too high, so we could not reduce costs this way. The option, however, was available, so why not ask about if this is possible for your parent? When calculating your parent's continued income, add the amounts of Social Security, income assets (e.g., interest from parental bank accounts), and pension earnings.

Worksheet 4
Researching Long-Term Care Facilities

Print a few copies of this Worksheet and rate each facility. Rate each point from one to five (e.g., one is poor and five is excellent). Feel free to note any additional comments you may have. If you feel uncomfortable or self-conscious about taking notes as you tour each building, take a few minutes to do so in your vehicle before you drive away so nothing will be forgotten.

If you are viewing numerous facilities, keep your comparison worksheets together. This collected and recorded data can easily be copied and sent to distant family caregivers for their thoughts and comments.

Care Center Information

Facility name: _____

Facility address: _____

Contact name: _____

Date visited: _____

Building condition and upkeep: _____

Location: _____

Parking: _____

Date of last building inspection: _____

Date of last elevator inspection: _____

Emergency evacuation: _____

Emergency lighting: _____

Lighting: _____

Cleanliness: _____

Room size: _____

Room shape: _____

Room location: _____

Staff and resident interaction: _____

Resident-to-resident interaction: _____

Initial greeting: _____

Staff experience: _____

Number of staff (both daytime and overnight): _____

Resident transferability within property: _____

Additional services (e.g., hair care, physiotherapy, nail care): _____

Medication lock-up: _____

Available amenities: _____

Religious denomination: _____

Resident activities (inside and outings): _____

Food and food service (consider menu variation): _____

Dietary requests: _____

Cost for care: _____

Visiting restrictions: _____

First impressions: _____

Comments heard from others: _____

Additional comments: _____

<><><><><><><><><><><><><><><><><><><><><><><><><><><><><><><><><><><><>

3.2 Limit the extras

Family caregivers often overlook the cost of additional services (e.g., haircuts, laundry, and day trips) provided through a care home; these are often not included in your parent's monthly rent. While there is certainly both value and benefits to be found with these extras, carefully evaluate what is actually necessary. Can you (or another family member) do your parent's laundry? Could a haircutting student come in to style your parent's hair at a reduced price to gain experience?

3.3 Invest in yourself

Hiring outside help, at any level, for your mother or father comes at a cost and that cost is likely to rise over the course of time. Instead of continuing to pay, you could consider taking on those jobs. Bringing in help can free up your time. A housekeeper, for example, could tackle your parent's household chores while you could attend to other matters. Carefully weigh the alternatives.

3.4 Call on community help

Are there community groups or organizations operating in your city? Contact each of these groups to ask if any of their members could join your own caregiving network. A member of a church congregation could visit and walk with your parent. A Girl Guide could read to your aging parent in long-term care thus providing a friendly face and mental stimulation.

3.5 Keep your job

While it can be difficult to both work and provide care, hang on to your job. While working does occupy many hours per day resulting in many caregivers reaching the proverbial "tipping point" and quitting their jobs to allow for more time tending to a senior loved one, it will provide you with a steady stream of income to afford your parent's care costs as well as your own — both now and in the future. When leaving your career behind, you are also leaving your own pension as well as other possible career perks (e.g., advancement prospects, sale bonuses, stock sharing, or additional educational and training opportunities).

4. The Future of Seniors' Assisted Living and Long-Term Care

What lies ahead for seniors' homes across the country? While I cannot forecast exactly, with the ever-growing number of American seniors requiring long-term care, it would make perfect sense to increase the number of care facilities available. We do need to address this problem now and not delay. Personally, I would certainly like to see this happen; however, my preference would be for an increased number of smaller facilities rather than more sprawling properties. The ideal would be to provide better individual care rather than just "filling rooms" and available beds.

A practical approach was taken by the Green House Project where residents have their own private bedroom and bathroom, but share a central living room, kitchen, and dining area in a home-like setting. With fewer residents (six to ten residents in each Green House pod) and far fewer staff required, seniors living in such buildings can greatly benefit by more direct care time (and better relationships created) from the staff who will not have to rush from one resident to the next. Green House management report its homes result in an improved quality of life and care, increased satisfaction of residents and family caregivers, and lower capital costs.

Bearing in mind the steady growth of the Green House Project (at last count, there were 144 homes available and 120 homes being built across the country and you can find at least one such home in 32 of the 50 US states), they seem to be onto a very good idea! To learn more about the Green House Project or to find a home near you, go to its website: thegreenhouseproject.org.

Based on societal need and public demand, it would be my sincere hope to see more senior's homes opening and operating sooner rather than later. Ideally, these facilities would be located in both larger and smaller cities and towns to provide increased access for all.

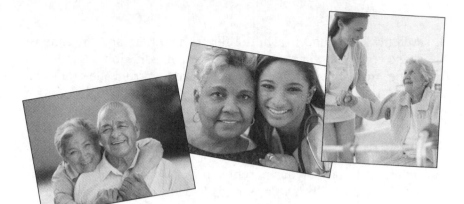

Chapter 4
Moving Your Parent

"I'm being uprooted," Dino said.

"You're being transplanted," Viv replied, "and to a better home."

– Stuart Woods, Unintended Consequences

When the time comes to relocate your parent to a new facility or long-term care, you, essentially, have two choices. You can either hire professional movers or undertake the job yourself. With a great deal already on a caregiver's plate, there is a lot to be said for the convenience of hired help; however, you must be careful with how you choose to move your parent's belongings. If you have the lead time, start calling around a month or so in advance. Create a spreadsheet to compare information, services, and costs. Find out if the company is bonded and ask for references. Will the company guaranty the move and reimburse you for any damaged goods?

When moving my parents for the first time, my sisters and I found a professional packing company to help us. Our parents' belongings were carefully packed and then shipped to us. While there was an extra expense for this service, paying for this was easily justified as it saved my sisters and I from the flights necessary and the time required to complete what turned out to be a massive job. As independent operators, this packing company saved us from the emotional baggage. Imagine how draining it would be to sort through your own parents' belongings.

1. Organizing the Move

If you prefer to tackle your parent's move yourself, expect an enormous job — especially if your parents live at a distance from you. As every situation is different, I cannot advise you as to just how much lead time you should allow; however, you can and should expect delays. This is Murphy's Law, which states that "anything that can go wrong, will go wrong." The following list should help you get organized and focus on what needs to be done:

- Gather ample, sturdy boxes for packing. Smaller boxes with handles are better to use so that you don't overpack and make them too heavy to carry. You can find boxes at your grocery store, place of work, liquor stores, office supply stores, and bookstores. Storage rentals and/or moving companies will often sell boxes different sizes (anong with other moving supplies). Start collecting these boxes in advance of when you need them. The best time to check businesses for discarded boxes is about mid-month to avoid the last-minute rush by other movers. Try to get similar shapes of boxes so they will stack easier and remember, when piling boxes, place the heavier boxes on the bottom.

- Acquire packing tape and a black felt pen for marking contents and room destinations on the outside of the boxes.

- Ensure that all your packing is completed before moving day. Pile all of your boxes close to the front door for quick and easy access.

- Donate, delegate, and discard. Downsizing is often necessary when moving a senior into long-term care, so you will need to find new homes for collectibles. If possible, donate extra clothing to a homeless shelter (call to ask if it has a pick-up service available). Donate the extra television to a friend who is just taking possession of a new condo or to your niece who may have moved into student residency at a local university. Difficult as it may be, consider discarding anything that is no longer needed. The hardest part of purging is often just getting started; however, you will often find a sense of accomplishment and relief to be able to see the inside of a parent's closet again.

- Call to rent a moving truck at least a few weeks in advance (whether you are hiring movers or planning a do-it-yourself move). If you are planning to relocate your parent at the end of the month, know that this time is popular for many other people to move as well and available moving trucks may be harder to come by.

- Double-check that your moving truck includes a moving dolly, plenty of furniture blankets, and a loading ramp. Don't just take the company's word for it — open the truck's back doors and take a look for yourself before driving away.

- Book elevators, if necessary, at both your departure point and end destination.

- Map your trip to make the best use of time. Would it be easier to move your parent first and then deliver excess items to a storage facility, or vice versa? Also consider traffic patterns to avoid any slow-moving rush-hour traffic. Are there any low-clearance bridges on your planned route that will be too restrictive for a large moving truck?

- Choose someone who is comfortable driving the moving truck (the truck rental company may insist that the driver be the same individual signing the rental contract). If you are uneasy about driving anything bigger than your own vehicle, take quieter streets to your destination.

- Enlist another driver to park his or her vehicle at your destination to hold a good space until you arrive with the truck.

- Be prepared for emotional challenges. Moving your parent into long-term care is not easy.

- Consider the expenses involved with long-term paid storage of parental items. If you can't find a home for your parent's couch or chest of drawers, or can't bear to part with something, the option of storing this may seem appealing. Make sure this option is financially viable for you and your family. Inside, heated storage (often preferable for electronics) will often be more expensive than an outside, unheated unit.

- Try not to adopt extra items yourself. I took a few parental belongings to help furnish my own home and to remind me of Mom and Dad, but I did not have the additional storage room needed for bigger items. Turning your garage, extra bedroom, or basement into a storage locker is not ideal either because you will be constantly reminded of everything, making healing and moving on yourself all the more difficult.

- Aim to complete the move as quickly and smoothly as possible. This will allow your parent more "settling in" time to his or her new home.

- Schedule your move during a quieter time at the new facility (ask the center's staff for time recommendations). The disruption of you carrying boxes in may confuse and/or alarm other residents.

- Exercise caution with what you move into your parent's new home. I was warned by Dad's facility staff that other residents may, unknowingly, pick up other's belongings, move them elsewhere and even hide them. This is a common result of dementia, but it could take months for you to find something! You don't want to risk losing a family heirloom. You may want to mark items with your loved one's name for future identification, if needed. Use a permanent marker.

- Confirm with facility staff what you can bring in for your parent. A small stereo system and portable television may seem like a good idea, but they might not be allowed as they could prove disruptive to other residents.

- Treat yourself following the parental move. Recognize your accomplishments by going for dinner or doing something special. Trust me, you will have earned it!

Now is a good time to also consider your parent's wardrobe that will be proper for long-term care. Looking good is one thing; however, a senior's clothes must be sensible. Considering a senior's reduced mobility and flexibility, shirts and sweaters should be buttoned or zippered, rather than pulled on over the head. For example, our family found Dad a warm winter jacket but the coat featured a double zipper. As this frequently caught in the fabric of the coat and wasn't always quick and easy to use, we asked a tailor for a replacement single zipper. Keep in mind that clothes fasteners should be simple for the benefit of care staff (as they will frequently dress residents). Following a suggestion, I purposefully bought Dad a few shirts that were one size too large. The extra room made it easier for a nurse to dress and disrobe Dad.

Also consider your parent's footwear. Velcro straps provide an excellent alternative to standard shoelaces. Pants with stretch waists can allow for increased comfort. Belts can chafe and be difficult to undo in times of sudden personal emergencies. Professional or office attire may have been necessary in your parent's working years; however, ties and high-heeled shoes are completely unnecessary in long-term care. Unless you are offering to launder your parent's clothes, label everything and ensure everything is easy-care.

2. When Your Parent Doesn't Want to Move

It's quite possible that your parent may not want to relocate to a nursing home. The first step for caregivers to take at this time is one of understanding. Such a move can signal further aging as well as physical and mental decline. For many of us, it is extremely difficult to admit we are getting older and are less able (or unable) to function for ourselves. We have likely spent much of our lives accomplishing things independently and it can be very painful to give that up.

A senior's pride comes into play here as well. Imagine how you would feel being unable to perform even the simplest of tasks like tying your shoes. This is something that you have successfully accomplished for many years; however, you may not be able to bend over or reach that far any more. When facing the need to ask for help with something, a senior may easily question his or her own competence and experience frustration.

If you tell a child that he or she cannot do something, that child will routinely try to do it anyway (and may try even harder to accomplish the task). Dementia in an aging parent can produce a childlike state, so expect your parent to try and prove he or she is able by doing something.

I remember hearing from the staff at Mom and Dad's home that Mom had been found halfway up the flight of stairs. When younger, Mom could easily climb stairs; however, she had become too weak for the eight flights in this building. However, she tried (unsuccessfully) to demonstrate herself able (to both herself and others). You may question similar acts and consider them foolish or even dangerous;

however, it is likely that your parent is scrambling for proof that he or she remains competent and in control.

While you may not want to encourage your own parent from attempting to climb eight flights of stairs, don't discourage active participation in the moving process. Cognitively aware seniors may feel fearful about moving into a nursing home. By looking ahead, a senior may be aware that a nursing home could be his or her final stop — death and dying are not pleasant subjects to think about.

Involve your loved one in the moving decision when and however possible. When touring possible facilities, invite your parent along and gauge his or her response. By providing him or her with the chance to physically view the facilities allows him or her the opportunity to meet the facility staff and other residents. Your parent may warm up to the idea of long-term care if he or she is allowed to accompany you on tours to physically see what such facilities offer.

As mentioned in the previous chapter, discuss the options openly. Does your parent have any objections, dislikes, and fears about moving into long-term care? Respect what your parents says and frame your comments creatively, such as, "I'm worried about you, but I know the staff here can take good care of you" or "With this property located so close, I will never be far away." Don't be timid and push the subject, if required. Your parent may be perfcctly content to have you drop the idea completely, but this may not be the best approach. Decisions may have to be made, and you have to press for action.

Granted, moving a senior is almost easier when he or she is not cognitively aware of what is happening. When my family transferred Dad to his locked Alzheimer's unit, he was in the late stages of the disease. There were no discussions and arguments. When a room became available, my sisters and I packed up Dad's belongings, loaded a rental truck, and brought Dad over in a separate vehicle. We did need to do some further downsizing because Dad's new room was just that — a room — shared with another resident and, other than a closet, offered very little in the way of storage space. The building also did not have any additional lockers or other on-site storage for resident's belongings. Moves can prove to be physically and emotionally demanding for a senior; however, in our case, Dad adjusted quite well to his new home.

3. When Your Parent Can No Longer Drive

When moving your parent into a long-term care home (or even before), it is a good time to discuss his or her driving. There are good reasons why seniors' homes parking lots hold more staff cars than resident cars. Rest assured that even without a vehicle, the senior will not be confined because the home may offer a transportation service (for a small fee) that can take your parent to and from events, shopping malls, and other destinations. Caregivers should note that seating on the facility bus or van might need to be booked in advance.

A person's vehicle can provide tremendous freedom and independence. A senior with reduced vision, hearing, or reflexes can easily turn their vehicle into a deadly missile. After a lifetime of regular driving, however, seniors don't always readily hand over the car keys or admit there is a potential risk. The convenience and appeal of driving can be great.

My sisters and I discussed the driving issue at length and decided that the best route to take with our parents was to show our joint concern. This was not a time to offer our help, but insist. Together, we approached Mom and Dad, voiced our worry, and successfully convinced our parents to give up the keys. While it was a very sad day when I accompanied Mom back to the auto dealer to sell her car, I was also very relieved.

Should your parent not be convinced by family requests, another option is to work with a family physician. Begin by booking an appointment for your parent — even on the premise of an annual medical checkup. Prior to visiting the doctor, call the office and explain your situation in more detail. If you cannot speak directly with the doctor, share your concerns with the receptionist to relay to the doctor. When you do bring your parent in for the examination, the doctor can now address the subject of driving and can urge parking the vehicle permanently. Doing this may seem a little underhanded, but, sad as it may seem, a parent will often heed the advice of a physician over similar advice from a family member.

Expect some disgruntled days and parental backlash. Having a vehicle taken away from you can be humiliating. Now is the time to introduce your loved ones to other means of transportation such as public transit, taxis, and seniors' driving services as well as family and friends. Why not explain to your parents that they can still get around quite well and be safer with alternative transportation? Depending on your their response, now may be the time to create some "make-work" projects to help him or her feel needed and valued. As an example, a friend of mine purposefully snapped a home furnace wire so that her father could have something to fix! This may seem a little extreme, but it worked!

After your parent relinquishes the car keys, you will be called on to run more errands and provide shuttle service. Take a look at your vehicle at this time and consider whether or not it will be appropriate and safe. The following include some things to consider with your own vehicle:

- Four-door cars are better for seniors as they are much easier to get in and out of than compact models.

- Avoid any vehicle requiring a high step to climb in as your parent will not be as supple as in younger years.

- A vehicle with a large trunk, storage compartment, or fold-down back seat (e.g., a station wagon) is perfect for carrying wheelchairs or scooters.

- Ensure that all required maintenance is done on your vehicle to ensure the most reliability for your increased travels. While you cannot guarantee that your vehicle will always perform optimally, regular service will help keep it on the road much longer. (I was once driving Dad to a medical appointment when my car stalled and refused to start. As a result, we missed the appointment, but my far bigger concern at that time was what to do with Dad. Fortunately, he cooperated by sitting in the car as I pushed it out of the way and then waited patiently until a tow truck arrived to give me a boost.)

If appropriate, you may also want to obtain a handicap parking pass to hang from your vehicle's mirror (the portable placard can also be transferred from one vehicle to another, if need be). Eligibility for such placards does vary, but many states will allow one in the case of various mobility devices. With the consideration of other drivers, you can park in reserved parking spaces closer to building door entrances making for a shorter walk for your parent.

Worksheet 5: Driving Safety Checklist will help you evaluate your parent's level of driving capability.

Worksheet 5
Driving Safety Checklist

Is your aging parent still driving a vehicle? If so, you have every right to be concerned. Part of your own caregiving job is to carefully evaluate your loved one's driving abilities and urge him or her to hand over the keys when driving becomes too risky.

Answering the following questions will provide you a time line as to when this becomes necessary:

1. Does your parent have reduced reaction time behind the wheel?

2. Does your parent struggle to enter or exit the vehicle?

3. Has your parent been recently involved in an increased number of accidents (even minor fender-benders)?

4. Does your parent rely less on shoulder-checking for other motorists?

5. Does your parent ignore using the vehicle's turn signals?

6. Does your parent drive too slowly or quickly for traffic and/or road conditions?

7. Has your parent recently received an increased number of traffic violation tickets?

8. Does your parent stubbornly insist that he or she is "just fine" with driving and blame other drivers for their apparent mistakes?

9. Does your parent try to turn on or off the ignition while the vehicle remains in gear?

10. Has your parent ever mistaken the accelerator pedal for the brake pedal or vice versa?

11. Does your parent ever get lost while driving on familiar routes?

12. Does your parent misjudge distances, such as between vehicles or when stopping for traffic lights?

13. Has your parent ever driven through a red light or stop sign without noticing it?

14. Does your parent appear more nervous when driving?

15. Does your parent tire more easily when driving?

If you have answered "Yes" to the majority of these questions, it is time to approach your parent, or have a family doctor do so, to recommend permanently parking the vehicle. Doing so is for the safety of your parent, other motorists, pedestrians, and you.

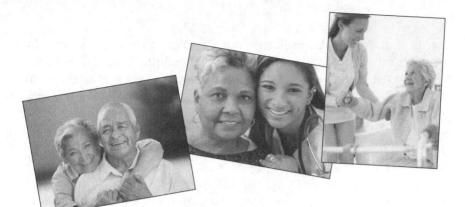

Chapter 5
Organizing Your Parent's Documents

"You can delegate authority, but not responsibility."

– Stephen W. Comiskey

Taking control of your parent's personal matters has to be one of the most challenging areas for a family caregiver. It is crucial that you keep his or her important documents safe and organized. It is also important for you to understand what these documents mean.

1. Keeping Documents Organized

When you are organizing your parent's paperwork, collect contact information for all of your parent's service providers (i.e., doctor, banker, financial planner, lawyer, real estate agent). Do not carelessly stack business cards on the kitchen counter or toss them into a drawer; find a better means of retaining these.

I purchased a small business card holder (you can find these at any office supply store) to keep these cards secure. Another option is to attach a cork bulletin board to your wall and pin the collected cards to it. When the bulletin board is placed by your home telephone, you can have all of these caregiving contacts handy; however, if you need to call or check in with someone when you are away from home, this is not as convenient. For this reason, I'd recommend programming contact names, phone numbers, office addresses, and email addresses into your cellphone. While programming can prove to be a time-consuming task, you are doing yourself a favor because you never know if, and when, you will need this information when you are away from home. In this case, know that many of today's cell phones have a camera. Snap and save a photo of each business card for your reference.

Effective and efficient filing systems can prove to be worth their weight in gold. As a caregiver, you will accumulate ample paperwork and you will need to store it. Until I realized I had to become better organized myself, I had papers and notes strewn about my home (even bright yellow Post-it notes framed my computer's monitor). When finally deciding all of this was not highly effective, I purchased a small, two-drawer filing cabinet and used different colored file folders to keep my parent's information easily accessible. As a visual person, I chose to use various colors of folders so I could immediately find what I needed; for example, there was a green file for banking and a yellow file for medical. With the amount of material I had collected, completing this job took several days; however, I was very pleased with the results.

Finding a few minutes per day to keep up with your filing may seem like an unnecessary chore, but it can save you immense time and headaches later when you are looking for a specific document.

In addition to long-term document storage, you may also want to create a short-term filing system of what needs to be done on a weekly basis. Using an accordion file, label each pocket with the days of the week. Slide your personal notes into each pocket; for example, Mom's doctor's appointment on Tuesday, her haircut on Wednesday, and parental bill-paying on Friday. If you miss an appointment, or if it gets rescheduled for any reason, it is simple enough to transfer your note into another daily folder pocket or keep it where it is for the same time and day next week.

You can also note these appointments in a day planner; however, I found that page space was often limited. Your best choice in a day planner will feature a "one page per day" layout; this will give you more room to write in multiple appointments. (**Note:** When scheduling appointments or meetings, resist the temptation to book things back-to-back as longer than expected line-ups, appointment waiting times, potential traffic jams, and even slower-moving seniors can delay you.) I utilized this practice and also paper clipped or stapled any accompanying information required (e.g., a business card with an office address, a dry-cleaning receipt, or a prescription notice to be refilled) to the specific page.

Your means of organization is only limited by your own preferences and creativity. A dry-erase board on your wall can be used and reused to note any upcoming appointments. An in-and-out basket can help you focus on what needs to be done and which jobs have been completed. For best results, choose the filing system that is right for you. Filing systems are not ironclad by any means; these can be adopted, streamlined, and/or discarded, as needed.

Some words of caution: While you will be collecting receipts, bills, and bank statements in your parent's name, do not hang onto such documents needlessly. This not only creates a mountain of paperwork for you to dig through, it also becomes a risk for identity theft. To best dispose of this sensitive information, buy a home shredder. Invest a few more dollars in a machine to ensure better quality. My first home shredder was less expensive and for a good reason; it very quickly proved to be incapable of handling the increased workload. Personally, I like the heavy-duty shredders that can also shred credit cards and staples as well as handle multiple sheets at one time. If your shredding does get out of hand, look for a mobile shredding company in your city or town. In my area, a fully equipped shredding truck can come to my home for document destruction. Maybe your banker, accountant, or lawyer could be convinced to provide safe disposal.

Worksheet 6: Document Organizer will help you gather all the information you need.

2. Understanding the Important Documents

It is not enough for you to know where your parent's important documents are, you must understand what these documents are about.

Worksheet 6
Document Organizer

Take a few minutes to complete the following worksheet to keep your parent's vital personal information handy. Provide photocopies of this list to your siblings. Store your own copy of this list in a secure place such as your home safe.

Parent's complete name: _____

Maiden name: _____

Nickname(s): _____

Social Security Number: _____

Birth date: _____

Birth place: _____

Current age: _____

Citizenship status: _____

Languages spoken: _____

Military status: _____

Bank(s) address(es): _____

Bank phone number(s): _____

Bank account number(s) (Don't forget any possible foreign accounts.): _____

Financial holdings: _____

Investments: _____

Sources of income (e.g., pension, savings, royalty checks): _____

Amount of regular pension checks: _____

Find the following information and obtain originals of these documents or, at least, know where to find them:

Driver's license number: _____

Birth certificate: _____

Marriage license(s): _____

Divorce record(s): _____

Property titles (both real estate and land): _____

Insurance policies (e.g., life, home owner's, health): _____

Tax records: _____

Will: _____

Advance Directive: _____

Credit card(s): _____

Personal property of significance/value (e.g., vehicles, coins, musical instruments, art):

_____

Personal debts: _____

Balance owing on each debt: _____

Additional contacts (e.g., doctor, pharmacist, lawyer, financial planner): _____

_____

◇◇◇

2.1 Last Will and Testament

It is crucial for you to know where your parent's will is located. Possible storage locations could include your parent's lawyer's office, a bank safety deposit box, or somewhere in your parent's home.

You will need to find out if the will is up-to-date and properly witnessed. Ascertain whether your parent was of sound mind when he or she signed it. Know and understand that a will can be changed and updated for any number of reasons such as your parent may have remarried or divorced, had another child, a beneficiary died, or the value of the estate substantially improved or became worse. Any, or all, of these factors can lead to the will being changed.

It is also vital that you have accessed the most current, properly executed version of your parent's will, as this will void any earlier wills that have been created. If changes are desired or necessary with this document, it can be best to have a completely new will created (rather than including handwritten notes or striking out sections of the text). If you cannot find your parent's will, or it simply does not exist, encourage your parent to consult with a lawyer who specializes in wills to have one created (the sooner the better).

Many caregivers use safety deposit boxes to lock away the important documents; however, you could invest in a small, fireproof home safe. You can often find a suitable model at your nearest office supply store or hardware store. You can also use the safety deposit box or safe to store other important paperwork including your parent's personal medical records, insurance coverage, birth certificate, passport, and home ownership papers. For the sake of convenience and keeping items together, you can use your safe or safety deposit box to keep other items (e.g., photos, extra keys) secure.

2.2 Living will

Unlike a final will, the living will (also known as advance directives) outlines a person's care and treatment preferences before death, should he or she somehow be unable to share these requests.

It upset me greatly to read my parents' living wills. Even though I was uncomfortable reading this information, my knowing, valuing, and accepting my parents' final wishes was vital. I may have been asked at any time to be a spokesperson for either my mother or my father. I know that both my parents deeply respected quality of life and felt if they could not "meaningfully contribute" in some manner, neither of them wanted to be kept alive via medical or artificial means. Fair enough, their request made perfect sense, but it weighed heavily on me many times. Fortunately, I was never called on to make one of life's most difficult decisions and stop treatment; I truly do not know if I ever could have done this.

2.3 Guardianship

When your parent becomes older, he or she often becomes less able to make independent decisions. In this case, family members can be appointed through the court to serve as guardians. As guardians, caregivers can legally make "life" decisions for a dependent adult (e.g., who can care for the parent).

Guardianship can be a complicated process involving a great deal of paperwork and it is best to ensure that everything is done correctly. Therefore, caregivers should consult with a lawyer specializing in guardianship before proceeding.

2.4 Trusteeship

Another role that caregivers may become familiar with is that of a trustee for a dependent adult. Similar to guardianship, a trustee is a family member or friend entrusted to make financial decisions for a dependent adult (e.g., paying bills, managing investments).

As with guardianship, this is a court-appointed position and potential trustees should consult with a lawyer for more information.

3. Medications and Medical Information

Don't forget to organize your parents' medications and medical information (keep everything in one file folder or box). Caregivers may have to go to greater extents when searching for these details as seniors may see more than one doctor (including general practitioners and specialists) and may get conflicting medical opinions. In addition, your parents may not willingly or immediately share this information and/or their personal medical details with you either as this can be a very sensitive topic.

Worksheet 7: Medical History Log and Worksheet 8: Medication Log will help you keep this important information organized.

Worksheet 7
Medical History Log

Copies of this important information should also be distributed amongst siblings.

Medical History

Family doctor's name: _____

Family doctor's clinic name: _____

Family doctor's clinic address: _____

Family doctor's clinic phone number: _____

Current medical condition(s): _____

Blood type: _____

Family health issues: _____

Allergies: _____

Previous major operations: _____

Dates of operations: _____

Injuries: _____

Date of most recent complete physical exam: _____

Alternate treatments sought (e.g., massage, Reiki): _____

Peculiar symptoms noted and dates: _____

Pharmacist Contact Information

Pharmacist's name: _____

Pharmacy address: _____

Pharmacy phone number: _____

Dental History

Dentist's name: _____

Dentist's address: _____

Dentist's phone number: _____

Date of most recent dental work: _____

Reason for most recent dental work: _____

Worksheet 8
Medication Log

With this worksheet, you can record and track your parent's medication history. Pay careful attention to dosages, side effects, and responses. This information will be very useful to doctors and care staff you may encounter. Should you have any questions, consult with your doctor or seek a second medical opinion.

Name of medication: _____

Prescribing doctor: _____

Date of prescription: _____

Reason for prescription: _____

New, temporary, or ongoing prescription: _____

Dosage: _____

Dosage increases and decreases: _____

Special instructions (e.g., take with food): _____

Side effects: _____

Responses (is medication effective or ineffective?): _____

Name of medication: _____

Prescribing doctor: _____

Date of prescription: _____

Reason for prescription: _____

New, temporary, or ongoing prescription: _____

Dosage: _____

Dosage increases and decreases: _____

Special instructions (e.g., take with food): _____

Side effects: _____

Responses (is medication effective or ineffective?): _____

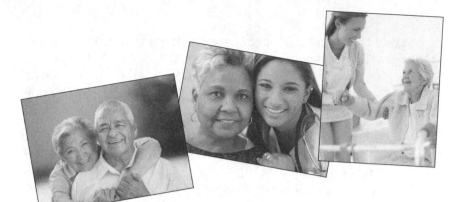

Chapter 6
Visiting Day

"It's not about how much time you spend together; it's about what you do with the time together."

– Unknown

How often you visit your parent in long-term care is your choice; as often as possible is best, as I learned. Hard as it can be to face or to admit, your parent may not have long to live and the final months will be your last chance to spend meaningful parent-child time.

While long-term care centers are becoming more welcoming, you may remain uncomfortable with visiting. Despite this, your parent can still greatly benefit from the socialization — and so can you.

Should you feel hesitant or uneasy about visiting, consider doing this for your parent's benefit. Imagine if you were confined to an institution or, worse yet, a hospital bed where you could not move; think of how welcome a friendly face would be. Would your mood not dramatically improve? If nothing more, you could sit beside a hospital bed and hold your parent's hand to share love. Even after Dad lost his ability to speak, I visited, spent time with him, and maintained a connection with him.

A good friend of mine once shared with me that he chose not to see his grandmother in long-term care as it was simply too painful for him to see her in that condition — understandable but unfortunate. As things turned out, she lived for two more years and he now accepts that not going to see her was a huge mistake on his part.

With routinely visiting my father, I became well-known to the care staff at his facility. They regularly complimented my diligence and pointed out a number of other residents who — regrettably — did not receive such attention. The reduced social interaction made these other residents easy to pick out — they were withdrawn and sat slumped over in their wheelchairs.

Another reason to visit is being able to personally monitor the daily care regimen of your loved one. Thinking back, I held, and still do hold, the utmost respect for my father's care staff, and seeing them work with Dad provided me with increased peace of mind. They were far more capable than I would ever have been and I knew that Dad was in good hands. As your parent's caregiver, remember that you become a watchdog when it comes to your parent's care. Therefore, try not to be too regular and predictable with your visits; instead mix things up a bit to keep care staff on their toes (e.g., drop in at 10:00 a.m. one day and 5:00 p.m. the next day).

1. Enjoying Activities with Your Loved One

Your loved one's medical condition will largely determine what you can do with him or her and when. Have a backup plan for when you visit as what you may have been able to do yesterday may not be possible today. I count my blessings that Dad remained mostly mobile until the end so that we could take our regular walks.

What enjoyable and fulfilling activities can you do with an aged senior? When it comes to planning these times, think of what your parent previously appreciated and follow suit:

- Can you take him or her outside in a wheelchair or for short walk around the block to soak in the sunshine?

- Can you read a story to him or her?

- Can you watch a travel video featuring a favorite destination?

- Can you listen to music or join a sing-along?

- Can you bring your dog or cat to share some unconditional love?

When it comes to possible activities, think outside the box, too. A neighbor of my father's in long-term care had his room walls plastered, from floor to ceiling, with family photographs. This way, he was continually surrounded by familiar faces and sights.

Can you enlist your loved one's help with folding laundry? This suggestion may seem a little strange; however, I learned that even when the mind has forgotten, an individual with Alzheimer's disease can still perform routine functions with his or her hands. You could bring in a laundry basket of towels and ask Mom or Dad to help you fold these; this will make for light work but offer a chance for you to talk with him or her. When the basket is done, explain that you are putting them away and leave the room for a few minutes. When you are gone, toss the towels around in the basket and return with "another load."

Some other creative ideas for your visit could include the following:

- Pack a picnic lunch and include a brightly colored picnic blanket.
- Play a simple card game. You can purchase an electric card-shuffling machine, which can make shuffling cards easier for your parent.
- Roll out a practice putting green (use a plastic golf club).
- Try bowling with a plastic bowling ball and pins.
- Plant or tend to flowers inside your parent's room.
- Write joint letters to family and friends.
- Finger paint.

Dad's facility staff organized regular field trips for residents where family members could go along. Can you join these field trips? If so, they can make for good memories for both you and your parent.

Common games can be adapted for those in wheelchairs. Can your parent toss a sponge dart, play a game of cards, or participate in lawn bowling? One of the most creative recommendations I learned of was wheelchair dancing. Look for a dance school offering joint classes so that you and your parent can take part together. While Mom or Dad may be restricted to a wheelchair, you should assess activities depending on what he or she *can do* rather than what he or she *cannot do*.

Depending on your parent's condition, perhaps he or she can still participate in an outdoor activity. While my father's mind was sliding, he remained in good physical shape in his later life. Knowing Dad's fondness for sport and the great outdoors, we took him to a local ski hill and had him sized for rental ski equipment, but we had no idea of what to expect. While our local hill paled in comparison to a mountain slope, Dad, much to our family's delight, smoothly and confidently rode the T-bar up the hill and swooped back down, carving huge turns in the snow; I had to ski fast just to keep up with him!

Keep in mind not just activities but also other comforts your loved one might not have access to within the facility. My father always was a great fan of coffee (he liked to say that he preferred it "hot as hell, black as mud, and sweet as love") so I began the habit of stopping by a coffee shop on my way over to pick up either an iced or steaming cup of coffee — season dependent. While Dad was always a little tentative with accepting the coffee, it didn't take him too long to eagerly and tightly clasp the cup with his wrinkled hands, gulp down the drink, and smile.

You could always just casually talk with your parent. Although your parent is in long-term care and may seem a shadow of who he or she once was, this is still the same person who loved you, cared for you, and counseled you through your own life's trials and tribulations. If you cannot generate any further dialogue past asking, "So, how are you feeling today?" or "What did you have for lunch today?" (followed by an uncomfortable silence), then come prepared. There are several ways to do this.

Prior to visiting, you could slide a few old family photos in your pocket; if these are pictures of family trips, all the better. When you arrive, you can show these to your loved one with a verbal prompt such as, "Look at what I've found! These are our photos from our vacation to Disneyland. Wasn't that a fun time?" Aging brains may still remember such special family times fondly. Be understanding, patient, and forgiving if your parent does not remember all the exact trip details. You may hear the same stories repeatedly. Just smile and nod. Although I heard Dad's story of how Cattle Point (a visitor's site in Victoria, British Columbia, located near their home) was named more times than I care to remember, there are still times when I would like to hear him recount it once more. I learned with my father that it was more important to talk to him when I could.

Another idea to generate discussion is to clip some magazine articles. You may want to avoid newspaper write-ups that report on current news, of which your parent may be completely unaware. While your parent may not admit it, he or she could be silently embarrassed about not knowing what exactly is going on directly outside his or her home. Instead, choose stories of personal achievement or social values. Your prompt here could sound something like this: "I just read this incredible story of Erik Weihenmayer — the only blind man who climbed Mount Everest. Have you ever wanted to scale a mountain?" Do you think that mountain climbing would be frightening or exciting? Ask your questions based on your parent's previous knowledge or interests. Keep your questions open-ended because these require a more extensive answer than just a simple "yes" or "no." With a spirited conversation, your loved one could become more animated and enthusiastic to share with you.

Because of a senior's reduced energy and attention spans, keep your visits short and understand the difference between good (when your parent is lucid) and bad days. Try not to be disappointed or blame yourself if your parent was not coherent when you came to visit. Instead, accept it and hope for a better day tomorrow. The better days can be magical.

Another recommendation for visiting day is to interview your parent. Compose a list of questions to ask and use a small digital recorder (such as the one on a cell phone). Please remember to have the recorder or phone completely charged or plugged in. While I never had the opportunity to do this with my own parents (and, regrettably, never pushed the idea), I was once, as a freelance writer, hired by two daughters to visit and interview their father.

Try to perform interviews in a smaller, distraction-free room. A low ceiling reduces recording echoes. If possible, shut the door and tape a sign outside noting "Recording in Process" to reduce outside noise. Understand that your parent may speak quietly so try to situate the recorder closer to his or her mouth without being obtrusive. Identify the best times of day to interview your parent. Is your parent more alert in the morning, for example? If so, you will likely get more detailed and complete answers to your questions at this time. Exercise patience here as you may hear the same stories repeated and, depending on your loved one's memory, facts may change. If you catch any verbal slip-ups during your conversations, resist the urge to correct your parent. If you are dealing with Alzheimer's or some other dementia, it will be pointless to argue as it will only frustrate you both.

Realize that you will never get your parent's entire life story in one sitting. Therefore, plan for multiple trips and, when discussing, help yourself and your parent by noting where you "left off" last time so you can easily prompt your parent with a gentle reminder about what you had been previously discussing. You can also bring a list of prepared questions to fill in during possible lulls in your conversation. When it comes to asking questions, don't be shy! Your parent may be flattered to be asked about his or her earlier life. With having these recordings, you will also have these stories for future generations.

2. Finding the Best Time to Visit

While family caregivers are often allowed 24-hour access to their loved one, you may have to adjust your visiting schedule to accommodate your parent. If he or she likes to take a regular mid-afternoon nap, this is not the best time to visit. Personally, when I found Dad napping, I always let him sleep.

Mealtimes, when care staff are trying to feed residents, can be very hectic; your presence may be more of a hindrance rather than a help. If your parent has any regular appointments with care staff (e.g., haircut, pedicure, or physiotherapy appointment), you may want to find out that schedule so you don't intrude at those times. I learned that Dad was bathed on Sundays, which is something I couldn't and didn't want to interrupt! Ask your parent's care staff for recommendations as to the best visiting times.

For your best visiting experience, look for a private place where you and your parent can spend quality time together. Long-term care centers can be busy places and not usually conducive to quiet family time. Is there a private visiting room on-site? If so, ensure this will be available at your scheduled time. If there is no such space available, why not make the recommendation to care-center management to incorporate such a room?

With our Sunday family dinners, we began by booking a small room on the third floor (we had to get our names in early in the week as this room proved to be popular). It was a simple matter to close the door to shut out most of the noise and commotion from outside.

Unfortunately, this room eventually proved to be quite cramped for our purposes so we eventually had to look elsewhere for a spot to dine with Dad.

3. Celebrating Holidays and Birthdays

Birthdays and holidays can remain very significant for many people as they age. Don't come empty-handed. Bring along a birthday or Christmas present. Choosing something may seem difficult for someone in long-term care because you are not sure what the person may need or what will be suitable. Understand that your parent will be appreciative for any number of things — your thinking practically will be the best. The following are a few ideas:

- Comforter for the bed. This will keep your parent warm at night and could add a splash of color to the room. If your parent already has a bed throw, pick up a second one to alternate when the first is being laundered.

- Slippers. Some warm and fuzzy footwear can be very much appreciated. Choose a form-fitting, rather than floppy, style for safer walking.

- Subscription for audiobooks. Aging eyes may not be able to read fine print anymore; however, your parent may still be able to listen to and enjoy a good story.

- Rechargeable razor. Personal hygiene remains important for your parent while in long-term care. Cordless models of razors can be used anywhere, so your father might use it while sitting on his bed or in a dining room chair. Empty the razor (and brush it out) regularly to keep it operating smoothly. However, be sure to keep the razor tucked away out of sight or bring it with you on visiting day. In my father's Alzheimer's unit, such smaller objects often could be mistakenly picked up by other residents and spirited away somewhere. Consider yourself lucky if you could ever find these items again.

- Home-baked cookies. Who doesn't like to nibble a delectable treat? Watch out for food allergies, though, and don't bring more than your parent can reasonably eat in a short time. Although having a few "extra" cookies around for later may seem harmless, these may attract unwanted guests (e.g., bugs or rodents) into your parent's room. Be aware that the smell of many food items (such as peanuts) can trigger allergic re-actions. Even if your parent is likely to consume these quickly, check with the facility staff to see if there will be any potential problems.

- Holiday decorations. Share some seasonal merriment with a festive wreath. You can hang this in your parent's room or on the room door.

- Small bookshelf stereo. Ask facility staff first before bringing any radios or music players because the sound may be disturbing to others. If such machines are allowed, your parent might enjoy listening to nostalgic CDs.

- Bathrobe. Choose a terrycloth style for increased warmth. As with all clothes supplied, make sure the robe can be easily laundered. While a colored robe can add some brightness, the dyes may bleed and damage other clothing in a community wash. To solve this problem, wash the new colored robe in cold water a few times separately before giving it to your parent. Tie a few knots in the robe belt to attach it to the belt loops — this will better ensure the belt does not go missing.

- Flowers. Brighten any room with a fresh bouquet of beautiful flowers. Not only will flowers color a dull room, they smell wonderful and will also improve mood. Recipients of fresh flowers can become happier. Place these in a plastic vase to avoid accidental breakage. Taking this idea a step further, why not "gift" a "flower-of-the-month" to remind your parent of your continual love? As with small food items, be sure to confirm with facility staff what is safe to bring.

- Massager. A little touch of heaven! As with the razor, look for one that can be operated without an electrical cord.

- Grandchildren's drawings. Invite youngsters to draw and color a picture for you to take to your parent. Completed pictures can be taped onto a room wall. Such personal drawings can hold special significance for your loved one.

- Family photo album. Supply your parent with a variety of pictures to look at.

Presents don't even have to be material to be greatly appreciated. Sharing your own company can mean much to a bed-bound senior. Having the grandchildren visit and sing a rousing rendition of "Happy Birthday" or a holiday song may bring a smile to your parent's face.

While I urge you to visit on birthdays and other holidays throughout the year, one of the most difficult times to see an aging parent can be the winter holiday season. So much of this time focuses on the family being together; when you visit, family memories may resurface and remind you that things have now changed. There are also societal pressures that people should feel happy and joyous (a hard thing to do when you are dealing with the physical and mental decline of someone you love). Old family traditions may not be possible anymore so it may be time to change these and create new memories. Know that you can still keep some memories alive and involve your parent in the celebrations, even if he or she cannot join you in the same way that he or she used to do.

One of my father's traditions was to read "'Twas the Night before Christmas." Maybe you will want to enlist another family member to employ the same traditions during your holiday celebration in commemoration.

The following are some suggestions as to how to make new memories while combining them with old traditions:

- Gather the family together and view collected photographs.
- String up holiday decorations.
- Share your stories; laugh and cry together (doing so can be very therapeutic).
- Experiment with a new gravy recipe, but use your mom's old gravy bowl with your turkey dinner.
- Continue to send the regular holiday family letter to distant friends.
- Tour your town or city and view holiday displays.

You could also create a new decoration; for example, use a small photo of your parents, frame it and tie some ribbon on it to make it festive. I remember learning that my father's care center honored previous residents with their pictures. I took part in a ceremony where I strung Dad's photo from a Christmas tree branch. By hanging a picture from your tree at home, your parent will still be with you over the holidays, even when he or she cannot physically join you. For another idea, family caregivers could also "reserve" a spot at the dining room table by placing a photo of the parent.

If you can, involve your mother or father in your own family celebrations away from the care facility. Remember that your parent may easily tire and a full day may be far too much to handle. For example, with my dad's Alzheimer's disease, he disliked sudden, loud sounds, which included his own excited grandchildren squealing with delight when they opened presents. We found it necessary to shorten his visits. If this is similar to your parent's situation, offer the quiet of your home's guest room to rest or schedule another activity for the grandchildren outside of your home (e.g., take them tobogganing or skating) so that your parent can enjoy some peace.

A few words of caution before bringing your parent to your home for the holidays — remove ribbons and torn wrapping paper from the floor (these can become tripping hazards), limit your guest list to only familiar faces and not strangers who your parent will not know, and don't have any unrealistic expectations for the day. What is most important is that you continue to spend time together — what happens, and how it happens, is irrelevant.

With an extended visit to your home, whether over the winter holidays or any other time during the year, remember to pack an extra set of clothes for your parent or keep clean clothes hanging in your closet. Should any emergencies arise, you will have something clean and dry for your parent to wear.

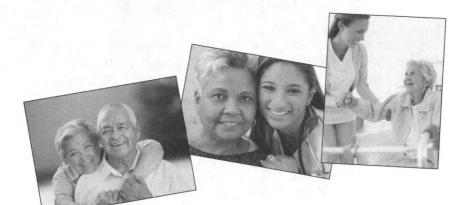

Chapter 7
Maintaining Harmony When Working with Family Members

"In times of test, family is best."

– Burmese Proverb

When you and your siblings are looking after your parents, expect some differences of opinion. You may not always agree on the same course of action. There can be mild skirmishes and much more serious verbal battles (to the point of family members refusing to talk to each other for years afterwards). It's easy for a family member to get his or her feathers ruffled when opinions are not readily accepted.

This should go without saying, but, if and when possible, you will want to remain on the same caregiving page with your siblings. Keeping things harmonious just makes sense as it is far easier to work and live with someone when you agree. Furthermore, important caregiving decisions can be made far more quickly and without delays.

When it comes to caregiving, however, maintaining family peace is often much easier said than done. Expect roadblocks or resistance from those closest to you. Others may feel that they have the best answer and will want to be heard and/or acknowledged. For the benefit of all involved, try to keep an open mind and maintain clear lines of communication.

Caregiving can result in both emotional and frustrating times. Your parent's health is failing and there may be very little that can be done. Tempers can flare without warning over the smallest issues. This may relate back to an old emotional "button" which could somehow be important to an individual. Caregiving situations can be emotionally charged at times. A family caregiver has not only his or her past and present to deal with; he or she may be already anticipating a bleak or painful future in regards to his or her parent's condition.

Sad as it seems, we humans also like to be right about matters. Knowing that we have made the proper decision makes us feel good; making that proper decision on behalf of someone else only increases our joy.

We can often take offense at being challenged with our recommendations. Therefore, when it comes to offering your own thoughts and advice to your siblings, tread lightly for the sake of future relationships. Try not to push your opinion onto others. Support your argument with solid facts. For example, saying, "I think we should do this" without substantiated information is not going to be enough. When you do make the proper decision regarding your parent's care, do not gloat. Nobody will like to hear this. Also, try not to raise your voice because it often makes a listener more defensive.

The best way to avoid an argument is by not starting one; although, this can be unrealistic. Once an argument has begun, one of the most useful tools to deflate it is through active listening. It may be more important for the speaker to be heard than to actually win the verbal war. Consider that the speaker may be venting frustration at the situation that is not even intended for you.

1. How to Conduct a Family Meeting

To begin, remove distractions from the room, pay attention to the speaker such as making eye contact, lean forward, and nod. Allow the speaker to fully vent without interruptions and then paraphrase for full clarity. For instance, repeat and summarize what has been said by stating, "I heard that you said ... ." Do not dismiss anything or harshly judge what has been said. If a point has been raised, it is important to the person who made the comment. In the case of numerous points being made, politely ask the speaker to prioritize these in order of importance.

You will want to begin each familial conversation by saying something positive. It is human nature to get immediately self-protective or defensive when we feel we have been targeted as having made a mistake or being wrong. Instead of raking someone over the coals, open your meeting with a compliment rather than a comment; for example, "I really appreciated it when so and so stepped in this week to … ." You may still face resistance; however, others will be more open to listening and conversing with you.

Similarly, if you are providing feedback on another's point, do so carefully. Implement the "compliment sandwich technique" of evaluating others. Begin with a positive affirmation or two, make your own suggestion for improvement and substantiate it with explaining how you feel things could be better, and then finish off with another positive statement. You are not completely burying the negatives; you are simply sharing them in a softer manner and communication will be far more pleasant.

Another useful idea is to plan to keep your own family meetings brief. By paying attention to the clock, your conversations will become more productive. Depending on the time you and your family have, try to focus on a few key issues during your meetings. By deliberating on just one or two caregiving issues at a time, you will be better able to give each topic the utmost attention it deserves. Draft an agenda for your meetings and indicate how long you plan to discuss each point; this will keep you more on track and help focus your siblings on the priorities.

The most productive meetings often list the maximum amount of time to be spent on each agenda point. Use a timer, set an alarm for each point and, after the allotted time, table the discussion, and move on. If a problem does not have to be addressed immediately, postpone the conversation until a better time, table a topic, or take small steps towards resolving it. Using these approaches can often be more effective than tackling the entire issue head-on. If you have ever made a New Year's resolution, you will know that you can become far more successful making a smaller promise, which makes the larger goal much more attainable. Unless an issue requires your family's immediate attention, stall your discussions for a day or so. Concentrate on pressing matters first and don't get sidetracked by more trivial points.

Agree to discuss these matters at a later time and date when everybody can return to the deliberating table with clearer heads.

Recognize the time of day. Later discussions can lead to arguments because people are tired and need to sleep. Appreciate that a brother or sister may have worked a long day or may have an early meeting the next morning. Emotions and worry regarding getting up in the morning can run even higher at this time. It is highly unlikely that you will solve any problems when you are exhausted. In fact, you are not doing yourself any favors or anybody else by not getting some rest and then returning to those issues the next day.

If your family has the benefit of time before a decision must be made, by all means, take as much time as you need. One highly effective problem-resolution tool is to brainstorm possible answers and take a few days to mull over these ideas. This often allows an individual to come back with a fresh, complete, and often better perspective. For example, with my own writing, I always appreciate "breathing time" before a project deadline. The easiest way to attain this is by starting an assignment early and adhering to a writing schedule. Upon completion, I can set the project aside for a day or so and then return to it with increased vigor and a "fresh set of eyes" to pick out grammatical mistakes or to revise a sentence or two for better clarity.

If you and your siblings live apart, alternate these meetings between your homes. Doing so may provide more neutral ground and may level the playing field. Also, try to hold conversations without barriers (e.g., a desk or a coffee table) between you. You do not want to appear oppositional during these discussions. If you expect these discussions to become heated, appoint a moderator (someone who is mutually agreed upon and respected) to help keep things under control. If possible, assign someone as the note-taker. This way you can distribute copies of what was said, and you can also review past conferences before proceeding, thus saving a great deal of time.

No matter what you speak of with your siblings, among the most contentious issues will be your parent's will and any potential inheritances. Depending on individual circumstances, even the closest of siblings can bicker about this. The anticipated monies, property splitting, or heirloom dividing can drive a wedge between brothers and sisters — a wedge so large that it may temporarily, or even permanently, alienate and completely separate family members from ever speaking to each other in the future.

In my opinion, it is best for all monies to be reserved solely for the use of the senior until his or her final passing. While a senior's future health needs are uncertain, long-term care can become very expensive. If your parent is of sound mind and wants to "gift" some money to adult children, this is another matter. Should this occur, you may wish to document the transfer of funds for everybody's complete protection. Do not consider any early withdrawals or creative loans against those funds. Although you may be looking at a sizeable amount of money, remember to make sound financial decisions based on what your parent would choose to do. While you will have day-to-day expenses and bills to keep paying, reserve the majority of a parent's accumulated savings for future health-care needs. Remember, health care can be very pricey and one cannot possibly predict what expenses are ahead.

When holding your family meetings, do not simply focus on the current issues. Look ahead. It is far better to be proactive rather than reactive with your discussions and responses. By discussing anticipated problems amongst yourselves, you will be better prepared. By learning more about your parent's health condition, you will have a more complete understanding of the possible outcomes. If your parent, like my father, has Alzheimer's disease, know that a secured facility will be required at some time so start investigating the housing options available. Will Mom or Dad require a motorized scooter? Will modifications be required at home? Do you need to clarify any of your parent's final requests? Please don't leave any of these decisions until the last minute or to chance. I have seen far too many caregivers (myself included) blindly ignore the reality of someone aging. It is far better to make those necessary decisions now rather than later. Reach out, research, and prepare.

Keep your conversations timely as well. For example, realistically you shouldn't have to discuss taxation issues until January or February. With the filing deadline of April 15, you will still have plenty of time to collect the necessary information. Are there more pressing matters that need you and your family's immediate attention? Devote your attention and energies where they are most needed.

2. What to Discuss During Family Meetings

What you and your family discuss at these times will, of course, be dependent on your own situation. The following sections outline a few key areas that will be specific to all caregivers and their family members.

2.1 Finances and banking

Knowing where your parent's money is coming from, how much is coming in and when, and where the money is going to require some simple accounting. Draw up a balance sheet to confirm income and expenditures. Create a spreadsheet on your computer and save it to your desktop. This will make it easily accessible when you need to record another entry. Keeping this spreadsheet up to date is helpful — especially if multiple family members are spending money on behalf of the loved one. In my case, my two sisters and I each applied for and received additional credit cards linked to our parent's accounts. This way each of us could buy something when required. For increased protection and/or security, apply for the minimum credit level required. Pay these bills promptly and resist automatic credit increases which can be offered by credit card companies.

Review your parent's financial situation regularly and go over this at your meetings. Does your parent have a more extensive financial portfolio including bonds, stocks, or mutual funds? Don't overlook the possibility of a foreign bank account, either. Your parent may also own property, antiques, and other collectibles which can increase in value.

Is there someone who is assigned to pay your parent's monthly bills? If so, that person may need to order new checks or he or she may want to arrange for payments to be made conveniently through automatic withdrawal.

2.2 Medications

What medications are currently prescribed to your parent? At the meeting, you might want to discuss each medication; for example, the time period your parent has been on the medication, dosage adjustments, and noted side effects. The discussion should also include who will be responsible for refilling prescriptions.

You will need to decide who will make the doctor's appointment and who will take your parent to the doctor to get the refill for the prescription. If a medication is required regularly, can the doctor arrange for an automatic prescription refill through the pharmacy? Even if you can get only a limited number of refills, it can save a caregiver time. Look into whether it is possible to set up an account with a medication delivery service sometimes offered by pharmacies.

2.3 Diet and personal care

You or your siblings may want to report at the meeting about your parent's appetite. If your parent is having difficulty eating food, either by holding a utensil or with chewing and swallowing, then some options should be discussed (e.g., buying specialized cutlery or chopping/blending food). Can someone talk to the care staff about possible solutions to these types of problems? Also, how hungry was Mom or Dad today?

Above your parent's appetite, observe how attentive care staff has been to your parent. Has anyone noticed questionable or irregular actions from the care staff? Alternatively, have you noticed actions from the care staff that could be commended? This may put your mind at ease, knowing your parent is being well taken care of in the care facility.

Analyze and discuss facility-care inspections. Is there ignored ice on the front sidewalk of the care facility? Does a chair arm or stairwell railing need tightening? Should a lightbulb in your parent's room be replaced? Is the toilet seat loose? Is a window stuck shut? Was the floor swept and mopped? If these areas are lacking the proper maintenance, you will need to talk about how to deal with these situations. When sharing these issues with care-facility management, remain firm but calm. Also, follow the correct protocol; for example, the home may require a written letter (if so, keep a copy for your own files to create a paper trail). Some issue you may need to discuss at a monthly care meeting with facility managers and family caregivers, while other issues may need to be addressed immediately.

2.4 Parental quality of life

Although a senior may be bed-bound in long-term care, he or she can still enjoy a good quality of life. Essentially, this means that he or she will be as healthy and happy as possible, be able to meaningfully connect in some manner, and remain respected. Family caregivers should ensure that their loved one enjoys at least some level of personal independence — including personal privacy.

Some topics for your parent's quality of life may include sufficient support such as inside and outside care staff. Consider who these people are, how many care staff are needed and when, and what their experience is. Other topics include suitable medical equipment (e.g., walkers or wheelchairs), and necessary on-site services (e.g., physio-therapy, massage, exercise programs) in place and readily accessible.

Does your parent still have continued family relationships and social contact with friends? If not, can your group come to a decision at the meeting about your parent's lack of social stimulation? Are activities or recreational outings meaningful (there is a world of difference between spending the day at a local park or museum and being taken to a shopping mall)? Does your parent appear to be comfortable at the facility or are there obvious signs of discomfort or distress? Watch for poor posture, restricted movement, and pained expressions as clues. If your parent cannot speak, it is even more vital that you speak for him or her.

2.5 Responsibilities

You might want to revisit everybody's assigned caregiving duties. You may find that someone is experiencing unexpected difficulty with his or her role. If so, you may want to delegate these responsibilities to other family members, outside individuals, or service agencies so as to lighten the person's load. If everyone agrees, you could rotate caregiving assignments amongst your siblings. This way, no one will feel burned out from doing any excessive caregiving task for too long.

The concept of amicably working together extends to many other individuals as well — specifically employers. Working caregivers can easily be drawn away from jobs to help their parents. During the process, they may face resistance from their employers for missing work, but working caregivers may not be as productive on the job. For example, I remember venturing off to work after a poor night's sleep and being distracted for most of the day thinking that my phone would ring with a caregiving emergency.

If you need some time away for caregiving purposes, talk to your company's manager or Human Resources department. You may reach an agreement to work flex-time, or unpaid work from home, reduce your work hours, job-share, or take a paid leave. Your employer may be willing to do some type of arrangement instead of being forced to replace you and train a new staffer, which can be a time-consuming and costly process.

With the country's rapidly aging population, workers dealing with elder-care issues while working will become far more commonplace. Employers have granted child care as an employee benefit — elder care is on the other end of the spectrum, but equally important.

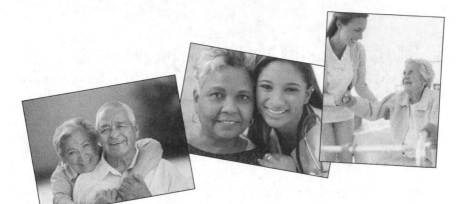

Chapter 8
Caring for Yourself

"To put the world in order, we must first put the nation in order; to put the nation in order, we must first put the family in order; to put the family in order, we must first cultivate our personal life; and to cultivate our personal life, we must first set our hearts right."

– Confucius

Whether you are just starting your caregiving journey or have been tending to your parent for some time, you will have likely recognized the incredible toll that caregiving can take on you. When it comes to caregiving, there is more than one individual involved — your loved one as well as you. Therefore, in addition to providing good elder care, remember your own personal care, health, and well-being. While the cliché of "taking care of yourself" has become very tired, think of your own needs in addition to thinking of those of your parent. You don't have to put yourself first; however, strive for a similar level to achieve much-needed balance. Doing so may sound selfish; yet, taking a personal break is anything but selfish.

1. Take Care of Your Own Health and Wellness

One of the most common caregiver complaints is stress. Stress is your body's natural reaction to dangerous or uncomfortable situations. When something unpleasant occurs, you can either fight, or take flight. Any number of issues can be caused by excessive stress such as insomnia, moodiness, increased susceptibility to sickness, and poor appetite.

When my parents were alive, I found myself incessantly worrying about both of them, although their health conditions were far beyond my control. I am usually easy going; however, I became prone to snapping at others. I noticed that I was rushing from one appointment to the next, often becoming far more aggressive and vocal at other drivers when behind the steering wheel. I also paced impatiently while standing in lines. I repeatedly checked my watch while waiting at appointments. Many nights, I did not sleep well. My appetite decreased, and on the rare occasion I was hungry, dinner was a frozen pizza, lunch the next day would a leftover slice of that same pizza, and breakfast would be a fast cup of coffee and a stale blueberry muffin that I picked up on my way to work.

You must remember to eat healthy and try not to rely on stress or sleep medications (either doctor-prescribed or over-the-counter). It is important to maintain proper nutrition. Convenience foods can be prepared and eaten quickly, and may seem like the perfect answer for busy caregivers, yet such prepackaged products are often full of unhealthy preservatives. If you don't think you have any time, prepare a number of slow-cooker meals and portion them into individual servings, then freeze them. One big advantage is that slow-cookers do not have to be continually monitored. Therefore, a caregiver can start a meal cooking in the morning, but still be able to run errands throughout the day. Defrosting each slow-cooked meal in the microwave oven only takes a few minutes.

Take a container of frozen stew with you to work in the morning, leave it on the staff lunchroom counter and the food will be thawed by lunch. Stock a bowl of fresh fruit on your kitchen counter. Vegetables (e.g., carrots, tomatoes, and peas) can make for quick snacks. Keep your top desk drawer at work stocked with granola bars or nuts for afternoon snacks. You could also involve your family members with meal preparation (and cleanup), on a rotating basis. Providing even one meal per week shouldn't prove to be too much of a hardship for anyone and this will lighten your workload and provide menu variation.

When you eat dinner, make it a point to sit down at the table with someone else. Doing so will encourage you to slow down and converse with another person. Turning off the television and ignoring incoming phone calls during the meal will also help. When eating, multitasking is not recommended. If you have children, you may discourage them from playing at or straying from the table until they are finished eating, so why should it be any different for you? Caregivers who are also parents are setting examples for their children by their own actions and they will naturally follow the lead. Yes, when I was a bachelor, I admit to eating out of the cooking pot; while this saves on washing another dish afterwards, it is recommended to completely set the table and use it for a meal. Wait until you finish your meal to check your email, concentrate on tomorrow's schedule, or read the doctor's report.

Before you rush out the door in the morning, ensure that you eat something nourishing. Pour yourself a bowl of cereal, sprinkle some berries or nuts into yogurt, or spread nut butter over toast. You'll find that doing this doesn't delay you excessively and you'll have far more energy to tackle the day ahead. In a pinch, grab a piece of fruit and tuck it into your jacket pocket for a snack later. Your body requires fuel to drive it.

Remaining hydrated is also important. Make sure you are drinking enough water for your weight and fitness level because it will help you stay hydrated and help reduce toxins inside your body. No matter whether you work in a high-rise office building or in your home's second bedroom, it's easy to keep a water bottle on your desk; just refill it as necessary. On warmer days, drink more frequently. You've likely heard the advice of drinking eight glasses of water per day, but, if you're like me, it's easy to lose track. Therefore, just keep a large bottle of water chilled in your refrigerator. Aim to drink all of it and refill the bottle on a daily basis.

Insomnia was a dreaded enemy for me and had obvious spin-off effects. When I didn't, or couldn't, sleep restfully at night, I was exhausted the next day. As a caregiver, I didn't know the meaning of the term "afternoon nap" and continually kept working at things that needed to be done. Being tired greatly affected my concentration and performance levels with work and school. There were times I would have to ask for someone to repeat a question or thought, simply because I had missed it. While there are plenty of over-the-counter sleep aids available at your nearest pharmacy, consider other, more natural options before you begin relying on medication to soothe you to sleep. For example, soaking in a warm bath or reading a good book just before bedtime can help you relax and leave the worries of the day behind you. Your own family doctor can best advise you as to the available (and recommended) options for sleep aids.

Options that helped me sleep included avoiding eating close to bedtime, using heavier curtains to darken my bedroom, and going to bed at the same time each night. I also experimented with a sleep hypnosis CD, which proved to be somewhat effective. You could also try turning down your heat or opening the window to allow your bedroom to become more chilled. Your mother's old trick of a cup of warm milk might help, as well as meditation or some relaxation yoga. Move the television set out of your bedroom because watching disturbing movies or news before dozing off will not help you get a peaceful sleep. If nothing works, book an appointment with your family doctor. Your lack of sleep could be due to a completely different cause. Sleep apnea, for example, can cause you to snore and this can actually awaken you from your own rest. If this is the problem, have your doctor refer you to a sleep specialist who may recommend using a Continuous Positive Airway Pressure (CPAP) machine for relief.

If you must have something to drink before bedtime, avoid alcohol. Instead, sip a non-caffeinated herbal tea before turning in for the night. While I briefly considered wearing earplugs to bed so as to block any outside noise and encourage me to doze, I realized that those same earplugs might also block the ringing telephone, calling me to immediate duty.

The problem might also stem from what you are sleeping on as well. Replace that aging mattress or box spring. An effective mattress should be firm enough to provide support (not too soft), yet still be comfortable. An older bed frame may also squeak whenever you move during the night, thus potentially keeping you awake. If cost is an issue, try oiling your bed frame joints, regularly flip your mattress over, and invest in a good pillow. Test your pillow in the store before buying it by bending it in half; the quicker it unfolds and returns to its original shape, the firmer it will be.

Furthermore, when the human body is worn down, it becomes more prone to sickness. While I'm no doctor, I fully recognize the importance of self-care for a caregiver and, even long after my parents are gone, I still preach this concept: "How can you care for someone else if you cannot care for yourself first?" Nothing is more vital.

When you are sick, you are little or absolutely no use to your loved one. In fact, when you are physically with your parents, you will pose a greater risk to them as germs may transfer. Remember, your parents and their neighbors in care facilities are much older and have weaker immune systems than you. If you are ill, this is no time to be visiting. You will be more of a hindrance than a help. I remember a sign at my father's long-term care home posted at the building's front door during a flu outbreak which read, "If you're sick, please visit us another day." Quarantine yourself until you are better. If visiting is imperative, wash your hands before and after your visit. You could also keep a bottle of hand sanitizer in your vehicle's glove compartment.

As a caregiver, you may experience bouts of depression. This is completely natural and nothing to feel ashamed about. While a particular disease may be out of your complete scope of understanding, whatever you can do as a caregiver is very much appreciated. You are only human.

We all have our limitations of what we can accomplish. For example, I remember a former employer of mine who slotted in his appointments at 15-minute intervals (in hopes of seeing more clients on a daily basis). We must realize that there are often extenuating circumstances which can easily delay us throughout the day. A potential client may keep us on the telephone with a few more questions, or a train crossing the road can stop us and result in our not reaching the office on-time.

Driving and talking on a cell phone simultaneously is another example of sheer foolishness. When you try to concentrate on holding a conversation and the steering wheel at the same time, the results can be tragic. As a caregiver, you cannot dart into the nearest telephone booth to change into your "superhuman" costume! With doing whatever is possible, you are remaining realistic as well as helping yourself, the care staff involved, and your loved one.

When I found myself bottling up my feelings, I compared myself to a volcano: I could erupt with little notice. To better explain, bottling up concerns and emotions may lead a person to blow up in anger at the most inopportune moments and at someone who may not understand the situation. Realize that both male and female caregivers will experience similar types of stress; however, they will respond to this stress in much different manners. Find a healthy outlet to reduce the stress. While I never found a support group strictly for male caregivers, I did ensure I found other means to relax and release negative thoughts. I shared my concerns with my sisters, I went to the gym, and I went for long walks to clear my head.

While caregiving is not all turmoil, you must find something that works for you as an escape. You cannot burn the candle at both ends before the candle burns through (a tired cliché but it is very true). Self-care for caregivers is not selfish. Take some time for you and never feel guilty for doing so. With your feeling obligated to provide care for an aging loved one and thinking that others may not completely understand your desire to break away occasionally, this is far easier said than done; however, you will retain your own sanity and not become a martyr.

One of the best things you can do for yourself and for your loved one is to watch for your own signs of stress or other unusual reactions. Pay attention to others' remarks that you may be acting out of the ordinary. Monitor these observations and record them on paper so you will not forget them. Are you hearing the same comments from different people? If so, these will not be just passing comments but actual concerns. If things become unbearable, see your family doctor for a medical diagnosis. Take your notes with you so you will have something to refer to.

If you think of a car, it can only go so far without fuel and regular maintenance. To prevent yourself from experiencing any flat tires or overheating and requiring a major service overhaul, learn to walk away from caregiving occasionally. Book a personal tune-up. Aim to release yourself partially or totally from your caregiving responsibilities. You will come back stronger and more revitalized. Don't you always feel better after getting a good night's rest? Caregiving can be physically, emotionally, and mentally draining and, as a human being, you simply cannot function forever without taking a rest.

2. Socialize and Pursue Hobbies

Your own self-care can involve socialization with others. Remember your friends; go meet someone for a cup of coffee and try to discuss matters other than your own caregiving experiences. Involve your friends when and wherever possible. Your friends care about you and want to help; however, they may not know exactly what you need. Friends can be a tremendous support through offering a sympathetic ear or a helping hand when you need it the most.

How you find personal respite is only limited to your own imagination. Examples of ways to take a break may include the following:

- Pursue a hobby.
- Explore a new interest.
- Register in a class.
- Go for a walk (if it is too cold outside, go to the gym and walk on a treadmill or track).
- Do something special with your significant other.
- Go to a concert.
- Book a massage.
- Wander through a museum or an art gallery.
- Volunteer.
- Go for a long drive.
- Don a pair of headphones and listen to a favorite musician.
- Watch a movie.
- Sip a cup of tea while reading a good book.
- Go on a weekend getaway.
- Take in a hockey, baseball, or football game.
- Head to your local mall and go shopping.
- Rake the leaves in your backyard.
- Clean your house.
- Organize a potluck supper with neighbors and friends.

As a freelance writer, I turned more to my craft for relief. I churned out many pages of stories and feelings. You can write too — you certainly don't have to be a professional — and nobody will ever see your journaling, save for yourself, unless you choose to share it with others. One benefit of writing is that you do not have to remain at home to do so. While every home owner in the United States is far more likely to have access to a computer these days, take a notebook and pen to the park. Pack up your laptop computer and head to the nearest coffee shop. Try writing a letter to your parent to say what has not been said; while this may never be read, the action of journaling and releasing your innermost thoughts can be healing.

3. Join a Support Group

While support groups aren't for everybody, they can provide an excellent means of respite for a caregiver. Support groups can vary in size and meeting scheduling and can offer the opportunity for caregivers to share in a safe and supportive setting. For a support group novice, a smaller group will allow for more individual participation and is often less intimidating.

While talking in a support group can certainly be beneficial, doing so is not obligatory; however, it can be good for a person to open up and share. Group attendees can listen, learn, and leave feeling better about their own situations just by knowing they are not the only ones in this situation. Often, there is no charge to join a support group and participate.

Look for a support group offered at a convenient time and location for you. Check for postings on a public bulletin board at your local hospital or advertised in a seniors' center newsletter. Remain open to the option of attending such a group with a sibling or a parent. Being in a sharing environment may encourage talking about difficult matters. If nothing else, information and other stories shared can be absorbed by each family member present.

4. Pamper Yourself

Pampering yourself occasionally is another form of caregiver respite. Give yourself a gift, because you certainly deserve it! These personal gifts do not have to be lavish or expensive. Of the many ideas possible, a caregiver will often most appreciate having some personal time. As a caregiver, you may not even realize just how important this time is until you experience it.

While it may sound insensitive, get away from your parent for a while. You do not have to remain permanently parked beside him or her. Think back to the times when you were much younger and your parents would hire a babysitter for you so they could slip out for a private evening together. They wanted and needed a break from parenting. It is no different for caregivers; you also deserve the privilege of a break.

Finding personal respite time over the holidays can become even more difficult. You may want to curl up and forget about the holidays entirely while others are hanging decorations and humming carols. With the heavy focus on the family at this time of year, it can become even easier to disregard or completely ignore your own needs. It is little wonder how so many caregivers can reach their breaking points and become more discouraged or even depressed during the holidays. There are also the heavy societal expectations to "feel festive" around this time of year, which is a difficult thing to do if your parent is declining due to poor health. Difficult as it may seem, try to remember the true spirit of the season.

For the past number of years (following my own parents' deaths), I have made a point to do something noncommercial over the holidays — whether attending a concert, donating a frozen turkey to the local food bank, or delivering presents for "Santa's Anonymous" (a local charity which collects and distributes gifts for needy families). Whether this is a new custom or an adaptation of a former family tradition, find something that works for you.

In addition, remember it can be okay to say "no" to a social invitation. Just because it is the holidays, you are not obligated to give your time if you do not feel in a festive mood. The same can be said for any other time throughout the year. I remember one previous year when I turned down an invitation to attend a work Christmas party. While there was some confusion and questions from my workmates, they understood when I explained my reasoning and accepted my decision. With that said, you do not have to be Ebenezer Scrooge — toasting the season with friends may be just the ticket to chase away your caregiving doldrums. Do what feels right for you.

Enlist one of your caregiving team members to look after your parent and some personal time just for you. Once I learned to release the caregiving reins and take a breather myself, I commonly escaped to a coffee shop where I could sip a tall coffee and read the daily newspaper. Your neighborhood coffee shop may be right for you, as well. Even an hour of personal respite time may refresh your mind and mood. Whether planned or impromptu, caregiving breaks are vital for caregivers. Find an activity you enjoy and partake in it as often as possible.

If you prefer something more material as a present to you, treat yourself. Go out for dinner at a nice restaurant. Buy yourself that suit you have eyeing in the store window. Book a professional massage. Any of these ideas can be enjoyed throughout the year. Remember to stay within your own budget. If your finances are tight, even a small indulgence (e.g., chocolate or ice cream) can make you feel better.

When planning respite activities for yourself, I believe it is important to keep them independent from your family. It will do you little good to sit down for dinner with your brother or sister as your topic of discussion could easily focus (intentionally or not) on what is happening with your parent.

5. Schedule Time for Yourself Regularly

No matter how you separate yourself from caregiving, book your own respite time regularly. Make a conscious effort to schedule time just for you. At the end of this section, you will find Worksheet 9: Scheduling "Me" Time to help you best manage your time. If this worksheet doesn't work for you, use any other means such as a writing a reminder in your day planner, making a comment on a wall calendar, posting a note on your bathroom mirror (or even on your vehicle's steering wheel), or setting a reminder for the same time each day on your iPhone or other electronic mobile device. It is far better to maintain and moderate your own health and well-being by properly looking after yourself, rather than overextend yourself and bc of no service at all.

Assess your respite breaks. How much more relaxed did you feel afterward? Listen carefully to others who may comment about your improved appearance and/or mood after your breaks away from your parent. You are looking for a positive report. By all means, try different activities to figure out what most effectively relaxes you.

To emphasize my point about the importance of self-care, I would like to introduce you to two real individuals I have previously met who took self-sacrifice to an extreme. First, a professional nurse, who, frightening as it sounds, continually refused to drink water. Her reasoning for reducing her water intake was that she would reduce her number of bathroom breaks, thus being able to spend more time with her patients. This same nurse also limited her lunch breaks and lingered after her shift longer than necessary because she found it difficult to allow someone else to take over. What changed her mind? When she became pregnant, she realized that for her son to thrive, she had to thrive herself.

Next, a gentleman, at a still young 45 years of age, went to his doctor with complaints of light-headedness, nausea, dizziness, and shortness of breath. The doctor's diagnosis was that this man had suffered from a heart attack and needed a triple bypass operation — not difficult to imagine as he was then tipping the scales at 400 pounds. His extensive girth was caused by years of improper eating and lack of exercise — examples of not putting himself first. Fortunately, the doctor caught this in time and this fellow wisely decided to make a number of dramatic lifestyle changes. Following open-heart surgery, becoming physically active, and changing his diet for the better, he reduced his weight by approximately 200 pounds and is far healthier and happier as a result.

Yes, you will want to do everything possible to protect your loved one; however, you must also protect yourself. Do not compromise on your own health. Despite a person's best intentions, caregiving can, and often does, become all-encompassing. It's very easy to get caught up with your own caregiving responsibilities and the daily needs of your parent, but by self-indulging a little rather than self-sacrificing, you will be a far better and much more effective caregiver. The more time you spend on caregiving duties, the less time you spend on your own family, career, and you. Remember to incorporate balance.

Worksheet 9: Scheduling "Me" Time may help you make sure that you take some time for yourself.

6. Delegate Some of the Work

In the world of caregiving, "taking a personal break" is referred to as respite. There are various ways you can find respite, such as removing yourself from the situation in one way or another or delegating another individual to mind your parent temporarily.

As a caregiver, resist the urge to try and handle everything yourself. You may feel as if you have a responsibility to your parent and may frequently say to yourself something like, "She's *my* mother and no one can take better care of her than me," but when taking on too much, you are doing your parent a disservice. Overloading yourself is unwise and unsafe for both you and your loved one.

When looking back, and even watching other current caregivers in my social circle, I will frequently compare a caregiver's actions to a trip to a buffet; the caregiver will often persist with loading more and

Worksheet 9
Scheduling "Me" Time

As a caregiver, please don't ever ignore the need for personal respite. You will need to remove yourself regularly from the situation to prevent things from becoming too overwhelming. Looking after your own self-interests is not being self-centered; doing this is self-protective. Use this worksheet to schedule some personal time just for you. Keep to this schedule as best as you can; you will feel better and more in control.

Activity: _____

Day: _____

Time of day and time required: _____

Personal rewards: _____

Activity: _____

Day: _____

Time of day and time required: _____

Personal rewards: _____

Activity: _____

Day: _____

Time of day and time required: _____

Personal rewards: _____

Activity: _____

Day: _____

Time of day and time required: _____

Personal rewards: _____

Activity: _____

Day: _____

Time of day and time required: _____

Personal rewards: _____

more food onto his or her own plate. As a result, he or she will either spill the food or drop the plate on the floor as it becomes too heavy.

Fortunately, in many towns and cities across the United States, you can find individuals and services to help you. To help you identify these resources, please refer to Worksheet 2: Your Circle of Caregiving (discussed in Chapter 1). Obviously, in a large city your network connections will be more plentiful than in a small town.

Do you and your parent a favor by easing up on your responsibilities. Delegate work to others. Let others help you. Remember you. Be kind to yourself and never feel guilty or selfish for doing so.

7. Find a Day Program for Your Parent

This is one of the many possible options for respite. My sisters and I found a day program for Dad. Twice per week Dad would be picked up first thing in the morning and transported to a local seniors' center. Here, professional and qualified staff would occupy Dad with games and physical activities throughout the day until he was returned home later that afternoon. We had to emphasize to the staff to keep their eyes on Dad as he waited for his ride in the morning and to watch for him to make sure he returned safely because his driver didn't always accompany him to the building door. This arrangement proved to be ideal for my mother who, at that time, was weak. With Dad away, she was relieved of her connection and the extra attention which Dad, unknowingly, required. Mom could relax peacefully without interruption, stress, or worry. Day programs are often advertised through local hospitals and seniors' associations; your family doctor may be able to refer you to some programs.

8. Interviewing and Hiring Help

Can you hire help? With the number of seniors increasing in the United States, more seniors' home-care-service companies are opening. This list includes major franchisors (e.g., Home Instead Senior Care and Nurse Next Door) who have office locations across the country. Company staff can tend to your parent's needs for a few hours and allow you some much-needed time and space.

If you have a nursing program in your area, you may be able to advertise for students to help you. Attending students may be interested in picking up a part-time job for the extra income and to gain valuable work experience as well as a reference.

When we were looking for someone to help with Dad, my family chose to place an ad in the local newspaper. Judging by our response, this proved to be very effective. We received a good number of résumés, short-listed our applicants, met and interviewed them, and then hired someone. As it turns out, our hire was a great choice, and remained working with Dad until he died. Place your ad in the weekend edition of your local newspaper to take advantage of the increased readership.

Probably the best way to find outside help is by referrals. Discuss with other caregivers what person or agency they would recommend. Understand that choosing an independent respite provider will provide your parent with security and consistency because it will be the same face visiting him or her. Note that a professional business will often provide you with whoever is available so you may never get the same person twice. However, there is something to be said for agencies having more staff so that you don't get caught unprepared. When hiring independent help, who can provide emergency backup if your caregiver calls in sick?

Should you want to hire additional help, it is best to personally meet and interview applicants. Résumés can outline relevant training, skills, and experiences; however, a personal discussion will give you a far better perspective on these individuals. When interviewing, note that you can only go so far with your questions; it is not permitted by law to probe applicants with personal questions involving age, religious beliefs, place of birth, political preferences, and so on. You are certainly entitled to ask for other facts. For interviewing purposes, try to meet somewhere comfortable for all parties and bring a list of questions so that you do not forget anything.

I remember participating in a number of interviews where my interviewer (or an assistant) took notes. Unless you are talking with a number of applicants and you do not want to forget any comments made, I would advise not to do this as it can be somewhat unnerving for the interviewee.

Design your questions be more of the open-ended variety to encourage longer responses (simple "Yes" or "No" answers rarely tell you much about a person or his or her character). Worksheet 10: Getting to Know a Potential Caregiver provides you with some questions that you can ask:

Worksheet 10
Getting to Know a Potential Caregiver

1. Tell me about yourself (this is a standard opening for many interviews).

2. Where have you worked before?

3. Are you familiar with _____ (name your parent's health condition)?

4. How do you handle stress and pressure (you may want to ask the person to give an example to get a better understanding of how he or she would manage in such a situation)?

5. Why do you want this job?

6. Tell me about a time you had to adapt in a difficult situation.

7. What skills have you acquired that you think would suit you for this job?

8. Would you be willing to undergo a security clearance?

◇◇

At the end of your interview, allow your applicant the opportunity to ask questions in return. Not only is this common courtesy, it will demonstrate to you how enthusiastic this person is to work for you. With initial interviews, you are not required to talk salary, but you should come prepared with a pay range you are willing to offer.

You do not have to make any immediate hiring decisions. By all means, take a few days to mull over the interviews, debate applicants with other family members, and call the applicant's references. You are making a decision which will greatly affect you and your loved one. After our family hired someone, we notified all the potential applicants (by telephone or email), thanked them for their interest, and filed the collected résumés away in a safe place, on the off chance that we might need to hire again.

You will want to confirm that your hired caregiver is physically able to safely lift and transfer your parent, and is trustworthy and dependable. Ask for two or three names as references, either personal or professional, and call these individuals to get their opinions.

If you are short-listing applicants and inviting several of them back for a second interview, you may want to involve your parent. Naturally, you will want to make those introductions before you hire, but you could evaluate interviewees on how they deal or respond to your parent. You will want to know this as your hire will be in a position of compassion, trust, and integrity. Welcome your parent to join you during this interview or invite your potential new caregiver to meet Mom or Dad at home. You will want to ensure that your parent is comfortable around the potential hire.

When you make the decision of who to hire, draft up a short written agreement in which you stipulate the hours of work and the rate of pay. Have all parties involved sign this agreement. To avoid possible intimidation, title your agreement as something other than a "contract." Instead, refer to it as "terms of agreement" or "terms of hire." Pay careful attention to outlining and itemizing the respite worker's exact responsibilities. Do you expect your new employee to prepare dinner for your loved one and do some additional housework? By fully describing the responsibilities ahead of time, you can help to avoid uncertainty or assumptions. Remember to date this agreement, provide a copy to your new hire, and file a copy for yourself.

As an employer, you will have a number of responsibilities to your employee. These obligations are listed on the website of the United States Department of Labor (www.osha.gov/as/opa/worker/employer-responsibility.html).

You will be required to pay at least the minimum wage; pay overtime (of 1.5 times the hourly pay) if, and, when, your caregiver works more than 40 hours per week; provide paychecks on a regular basis (mid-month and end of the month is a perfectly acceptable arrangement); and include a statement showing gross pay, deductions, and net pay for both the pay period and the year to date.

Employers are also responsible for withholding tax from employees and remitting these monies to the government on a timely basis. Your employee must also be kept informed as to how much is being deducted from each paycheck. Contact the Internal Revenue Service (IRS) for more information about employment taxes in your jurisdiction. To avoid a long and complicated discussion about state employment law, just know that these laws do vary. A helpful resource is the US Department of Labor's list of every state office and website address (www.dol.gov/whd/contacts/state_of.htm).

Until we found it no longer necessary to do so, my family approached the care staff at Dad's facility to verify that our hired companion arrived as scheduled. Be mindful when making this request as long-term care employees already have plenty to do. I also made several unscheduled visits to coincide with our worker's time with Dad. I explained that my premise for visiting was for some other reason; however, my main purposes for stopping by were to ensure that she was on-site and to watch how she interacted with my father. I also designed a time sheet on which our caregiver noted her hours of work, explained any outings and activities, and attached any receipts for related expenses for reimbursement. I provided ample space for her to jot down any of Dad's behavioral changes — even if I was not present to witness it, it was comforting for me to read that my father "responded well" and/or "had a good day." My family felt that writing this information down helped to keep her accountable while also keeping us well-informed.

9. Taking Care of Yourself after Your Loved One Dies

While caring for yourself during your caregiving years can prove to be greatly beneficial, caregivers must also consider their own future self-care. At some point in time, your loved one will pass away and your life will, once again, change. Many caregivers report feeling lost after a parent dies (either suddenly or expectedly). Remember that you have spent much time and effort caring for someone else so it is completely understandable that you may feel abandoned and unsure as to how you now must move forward.

You can help yourself dramatically by preparing for the end and learn what happens when a person dies. A doctor or a hospice nurse can best advise you as to what your loved one may experience before passing away. If you have not done so already, take some steps to learn what your responsibilities are. If your loved one has requested a traditional burial, select a casket sooner, rather than later.

Take some time to consider how you will manage immediately following the death of your loved one. You will likely feel alone, confused, and exhausted — especially in the first few weeks. You will also have plenty to do, such as arranging the service for your loved one, cleaning out his or her home, and notifying authorities and other interested parties of your loved one's death.

Focus on the "here and now" rather than any long-range goals. Planning proactively for this time will serve you far better than responding reactively. One simple question to ask yourself is: How will you best cope? Will you lean on others for love and support, or deal with it on your own? Choosing to be alone is fine; however, be mindful not to completely shut yourself off from other family members and friends.

Another step you can take to speed your own healing is to find at least one person you can turn to for support and direction. This person could be someone you know; perhaps a former caregiver who will understand what you may be experiencing. Leaning on someone who has already traveled the same road as you have is not necessarily burdensome to this other individual — many former caregivers (such as myself) enjoy helping others and find doing so very rewarding.

Alternatively, you may prefer to meet with a professional such as your own doctor, a church minister, or a qualified grievance counselor. Whoever you choose should be trustworthy, nonjudgmental, and available.

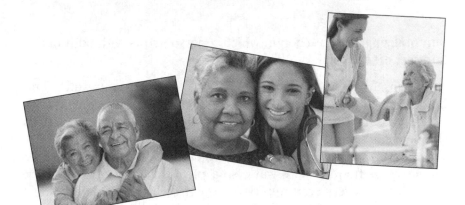

Chapter 9
Remaining Active

"Men must necessarily be the active agents of their own well-being and well-doing; they themselves must in the very nature of things be their own best helpers."

– Samuel Smiles

Caregivers and loved ones should always take measures to remain active because this has been repeatedly proven to promote good health. When I say "remain active," physical activity will jump to mind immediately for many. Remember, the human body is a machine and is meant to move, lift, twist, and turn. Keeping mobile also increases flexibility and circulation.

In my father's case, I recognized the need for physical activity and was strongly encouraged by facility care staff to take our regular walks. There were many other residents confined to wheelchairs and I wanted to do all I could to prevent Dad from ending up being strapped into a chair and being unable to walk around. Being restrained in this matter happens for a person's own safety because if he or she cannot stand, he or she cannot fall; however, where is the quality of life in that? Dad would have never understood being buckled in. Even worse, Dad might have ended up in a bucket chair — a demoralizing plastic scoop in which a person rests with both hands and feet off the floor.

Thankfully, Dad's nursing home accommodated our walks. The building itself was designed in the shape of a starfish where each of the building's extended arms was another lengthy hallway. When the halls got jammed with medical equipment or other residents or I got tired of the same scenery, I could easily take Dad down to one of the lower floors. There was also a pleasant fenced-in backyard, where I took every opportunity to visit with Dad. We could either loop around the yard until Dad grew tired or just sit in the sun.

1. Preparing and Taking Your Parent for Seasonal Outings

If you can take your parent out, but don't like or trust the weather, experiment with mall walking. Even in the most inclement weather, you can join others to stroll through a local shopping mall for both socialization and exercise. If you can, find a mall-walking group in your area. If such a group does not exist, take the initiative and create your own. Invite other family caregivers to join you, post signage at the mall, and check with your local newspaper to ask if it will print your community announcement on an ongoing basis at no charge to you.

As a word of caution: Heavy pedestrian traffic in a shopping mall can be confusing and possibly dangerous for some seniors. Drop in or call the mall's administration office to ask when the mall is less busy. Sometimes, a shopping mall is opened earlier for the benefit of mall walkers. Granted, mall walkers will have to be early risers to take advantage of this arrangement, yet without other shoppers milling about, this can be very appealing.

Shopping malls are not the only places where a person can walk indoors. I have seen many seniors at the nearby gym. While a few of the more spry seniors walk on treadmills, I prefer to see them circling the track as it seems a bit safer.

If you do walk outside on a year-round basis, an elderly person will require some extra precautions. Aging skin becomes more sensitive to the sun. In the summertime, have your parent wear a broad-brimmed hat to protect him or her from sunburn. Long sleeves, even in warmer temperatures, will also help to prevent burning plus reduce insect bites. Don't forget to carry along plenty of mosquito repellent and extra sunblock.

In the wintertime, bundle up. Have your parent wear mittens, as these are warmer than gloves. On the fiercest winter days, wear a lighter pair of gloves underneath a pair of mittens.

Choose a pair of winter boots for your parent that can easily slide on and off, offer stability, and which have a good tread for increased grip. A lower and flatter boot heal is also preferable and far more sensible. My family found Dad a pair of winter boots with removable insoles, which could be slid out and dried easily.

A senior's winter jacket should extend past the waist to offer increased warmth and have conventional fasteners. Keep things as simple as possible for both your hands and older hands (which can lack dexterity). Look for function over fashion! As mentioned in an earlier chapter, my father's parka, while warm enough, featured a double zipper. When the cold wind was howling outside, this proved to be much more annoying than useful as the zipper would often refuse to slide up or down easily and also get caught in the jacket fabric. It didn't take very long for us to get a tailor to replace the zipper.

Your parent will remain much warmer when you dress him or her in layers. As with the winter jacket, those additional layers should close with a zipper or buttons down the front of the garment. Crew neck sweaters, while fashionable, are challenging, if not impossible, for a senior to pull on. A material such as Thinsulate offers superb warmth without bulk or excessive weight.

When it comes to choosing your winter walking route, always stick with cleared sidewalks. Packed-down snow can appear to be quite safe; however, it can be quite deceiving as it may hide treacherous black ice underneath. Excessive snow and ice build-up can be immensely risky for both of you to walk on. If you fall, your parent will likely tumble as well.

While you cannot always prevent a fall, you can certainly limit the chances of this happening. One simple way to reduce the risk is with lightweight ice grips. Made of rubber and available in different sizes, these can be stretched over the sole of the shoe or boot to provide increased traction. With ice grips being quite popular with joggers, you will likely find these for sale at your local sporting goods store.

If your loved one is in a wheelchair or uses a walker, stay clear of the snow as this makes pushing and navigating even more difficult. You'll only have to try steering a wheelchair through deep snow once to agree.

Here are a few additional cold weather walking tricks so that "Old Man Winter" doesn't get the best of your parent:

- Pack along a small bag of cat litter. By sprinkling this on a particularly slippery section of sidewalk, your parent can get a better grip and far safer footing. If you don't have to take much cat litter, pour some into a ziploc bag with a secure closure.

- Walk slower and take smaller steps. While you may be tempted to rush from your car to inside a warm building, you are asking for trouble when moving quickly across an icy surface. Depending on your parent's cognitive state, he or she may not even be aware that the snow and ice has become dangerous. As a caregiver, you must take the lead. By hesitating and keeping your feet closer together when you walk, you and your parent can achieve better balance and be able to both stand and walk more securely.

- Experiment with a cane. A senior's cane can act as both an extra leg and an inquisitive finger. When using a cane, your parent can move more confidently on ice. A cane can also be used to reach out and poke at potentially threatening areas to ascertain just how safe these areas will be. There are also cane ice grips; these are small teeth that can be attached to the end of a cane and be raised or lowered as needed.

- Attach a pair of Yaktrax to your parent's footwear. These products feature rubberized bands to fit different sized footwear and studs which will dig into the ice and snow. These lightweight tools can improve both a senior's and a caregiver's confidence when walking on slippery sidewalks. You can often find Yaktrax at sporting-goods or shoe stores.

- Have your parent wear a belt. By grasping onto the belt (by the small of your parent's back) and holding on tightly, you will be better able to steady him or her.

No matter what the season, when it comes to walking outside with your parent, you will have to remain extra attentive. Watch for sidewalk cracks, uneven surfaces, and obstacles in your way. Even an innocent branch on the sidewalk can pose a risk because your parent may only shuffle along rather than lifting a foot to step over something.

Also, please walk with your loved one on the inside of the sidewalk, rather than on the outside. I am reminded of one day when I took Dad out for a summer stroll. While I was tightly holding Dad's arm to support him, Dad was walking on my left-hand side, next to the curb. I thought nothing of this but I accidentally loosened my grip on Dad's arm and he slipped and fell off the uneven curb. Before I could catch him, Dad hit the street, cut his forehead open, and started bleeding. While the cut was not serious, this caused me great angst. Fortunately, a kind motorist stopped and offered us a ride back to the care facility where Dad was bandaged up.

Whether you are going around the block or straying further from the care facility, stay to more trafficked routes and tuck your cell phone and a few extra dollars for cab fare in your pocket just in case. There are two important lessons here: Always hold firmly to your loved one and always be aware.

2. Find Time for Your Own Physical Activity

Keep physically active yourself. Personally, I've always liked to walk. Doing this doesn't require any specialized sporting equipment. I didn't necessarily have to have any destination in mind. Lacing up a pair of comfortable shoes and getting outside often proved to be very therapeutic. Fresh air and movement were often helpful in clearing my head and reducing my stress level.

You may prefer more intense exercise. I have advanced from walking to running. This initiative began several years ago when I was encouraged to join a "Learn to Run" club through a local running store. Completing this group with the support and encouragement of others motivated me to continue and aim for longer distances. If running doesn't appeal to you, join a gym. To increase your workout regimen, choose a gym in your neighborhood that you are comfortable with. Consult with gym staff about proper equipment use, exercise classes, diet and nutrition, and even personal trainers.

If you cannot find the time to go running, or get to your local gym a minimum of three times per week, look at healthy alternatives. Get creative with your ideas for "sneaky" fitness! Climb the stairs at your office building, park your car further away from the shopping mall door to encourage walking, take the dog for a walk, or do some heavier housework.

Try not to get caught up in the same routine either. I have several neighborhood running routes mapped out to offer variety. Running the same path or doing the same exercises will get boring quickly, and a boring exercise routine almost always gets dropped. Spice things up. In the spring and summer, you can go for a walk or run one day (include a few hills to climb), play tennis the next, and then go for a bicycle ride on another day. In the wintertime, your outside choices may seem more limited, but don't let the colder temperatures hamper you; take up cross-country skiing or snowshoeing, toboggan with your children, go skating, or swimming at the local pool (include a dip in the hot tub or a steam in the sauna afterwards). Enlist a friend or partner to exercise with you to provide both companionship and motivation.

3. Activity Isn't All about Physical Exercise

Exercise your mind as well. Don't ignore your brain's constant need to learn. Have you always wanted to study Japanese? Or learn how to make stained glass? What about a cooking course? Enroll in a class. Doing this will benefit you in two ways: Learning will stimulate your brain and provide you with a welcome distraction from your caregiving duties. Classes, workshops, lectures, and seminars can also provide you an excellent joint activity for you and your parent.

Read books on things you are interested in, in addition to practical information on your parent's medical condition and/or how to become a better caregiver. Pick up some books in your favorite genre. Frequent a secondhand bookstore or arrange a "book swap" with friends as a means to experiment with new authors cost-effectively. Alternatively, support your local library with purchasing a membership. When joining the library, you will get almost unlimited book-borrowing privileges.

If your bookshelves are already brimming to capacity and you don't fancy yourself collecting even more books, consider purchasing an e-reader where you can buy and store practically an unlimited supply of titles. These readers are light, compact, and slim enough to slip into a coat pocket, thereby making them perfect for on-the-go caregivers; you will always have something new to read when waiting at the doctor's office. Replacing and downsizing your own collection of books may be a challenge, but you can always find a home for good books by selling them to a used bookstore or donating them to a seniors' home.

With today's technology, you don't even need to curl up in your armchair to read. There are audiobooks that can be listened to in the car or while you are out walking the dog. Local libraries often stock a wide variety of audiobooks for patrons to borrow.

Spiritual exercise is also important to maintain an overall individual balance. Practice and live your own faith, if applicable, as you regularly do. Attend your church. Calm racing thoughts through meditation or try a yoga class or Tai Chi.

As a caregiver, remain socially active and urge your parent to follow suit. If your parent remains lackadaisical about going out, arrange for neighbors to visit him or her instead. While we may not always crave companionship, human beings are social animals who can enjoy spending time with others. Even a few words of simple conversation can make us feel better, more involved, and more mentally stimulated.

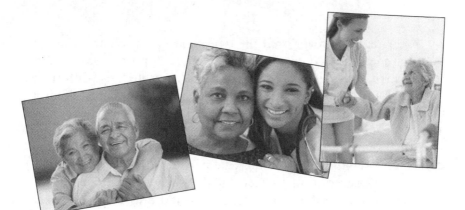

Chapter 10
Men and Women Care Differently

"Women eat ice-cream, men toast marshmallows."

– Dianna Hardy, Cry of the Wolf

When you look around, you will likely see that the majority of caregivers are women. You may fall into that category yourself. According to The National Alliance for Caregiving and AARP "more women than men are caregivers: an estimated 66% of caregivers are female. One-third (34%) take care of two or more people, and the average age of a female caregiver is 48."[1]

When it comes to caregiving, the job most often falls on a daughter's (or wife's) shoulders. Without wanting to sound stereotypical, women, by their assumed nature, are perceived to be more patient and nurturing and, therefore, can make excellent caregivers. Nursing schools across the country will, typically, see more females than males applying for programs. As a male co-caregiver, I was, therefore, more of a rarity, but men are just as capable of providing care for a loved one. Thankfully, this understanding is become more socially acknowledged.

---

1   The National Alliance for Caregiving and AARP (2009), Caregiving in the US National Alliance for Caregiving. Updated: November 2012.

Recognize, however, that the types and levels of care will differ between men and women. The two genders approach and respond to the job of caregiving much differently. Celebrate these differences and allow for caregivers to function where they feel most comfortable and are most able. Men can serve as a guardian for a dependent adult, deliver a meal, or drive a senior to a medical appointment. In my role, I managed Mom and Dad's bank account and investments, paid their ongoing monthly bills, helped move them (repeatedly), provided transportation to medical appointments and elsewhere, shopped for new clothes for Dad, and visited routinely. As you can see, the role of a caregiver is not strictly limited to providing personal care.

Without wanting to sound stereotypical (once again), men may be more firm when advocating for an aging loved one. If there is a family meeting scheduled at a parent's care home, men may be more likely to ask the tough questions and demand answers of the authorities. In her book, *Men as Caregivers: Theory, Research, and Service Implications*, Betty J. Kramer explains that "men in our society are often expected to be in control, confident, concerned with thinking than feeling, rational, assertive, courageous, competitive, concerned with achieving goals and tasks, action oriented, and able to endure stress and pain."[2] While men have long been painted as the "strong providers" in our society, it is important to recognize that men have feelings, too, but men deal with them differently.

Women are much more apt to share and communicate while men will remain silent and not want to readily admit there could be a problem too large for them to handle. I have often been described as being quiet. Granted, this is more so due to my introverted nature. I also cringe at the very idea of attending a "professional networking" event or even a friend's wedding where it will be expected that I meet and make small talk with complete strangers. With practice, these sorts of outings do become easier. However, being in the public spotlight and/or sharing my innermost thoughts and feelings (even with my closest loved ones) is still something I find difficult to do.

Men are the "fixers" and "doers" in our world. We like to tackle a problem and find a solution. If there is something that cannot be corrected, men tend to look at it as defeat (and we don't always like to admit this fact). When it comes to caregiving, however, the answer

---

2 *Men as Caregivers: Theory, Research, and Service Implications*, Betty J. Kramer and Edward H. Thompson, Jr., Editors, accessed April 2015. http://books.google.ca/books?hl=en&lr=&id=tvkKje6sMrcC&oi=fnd&pg=PA3&dq=male+caregivers+seeking+support&ots=GQT0Oj0sFm&sig=HbaWjG-m2q4ZApFI4TrJqM4Bz-j8#v=onepage&q=male%20caregivers%20seeking%20support&f=false

is not always as easy as oiling a squeaky door hinge or replacing a leaking kitchen faucet. Men do not always readily accept this but are not always willing to openly discuss their difficulties with the situation. Instead, a man is more likely to bottle up his frustrations and hide his tears. Men are, however, equally able to cry, but will often find more private moments to do so.

I remember seeing Dad cry when he realized Mom had died; however, he very quickly turned away from me, in a effort to hide is tears. If you are a male caregiver, please try not to bottle up your emotions. If you know a male caregiver, please try to get him to open up or vent appropriately.

If a man prefers not to share publicly within a support group, he may do so via an Internet message board. These websites offer users more anonymity for people to reach out to others for advice and encouragement. One key advantage is that users are not restricted to living in the same geographical area. Message board users are also not restricted by time and can ask their questions or read other's comments around the clock. Message board users living in smaller towns across the country can find this type of communication helpful as it offers a snapshot of resources available in larger cities. One drawback, however, is that the answers to caregiving questions may not be provided immediately. One can pose a question at any time, but expecting a prompt reply is not always realistic as other users may not log in for several days, be able to respond, or even choose to reply to a posted question.

Within a man's circle of friends, he will more likely have "casual acquaintances" rather than "close and trusted friends" to confide. Men are more often apt to go out for a few drinks "with the guys" than sitting down with them and having a warm, heart-to-heart conversation. It may be months between a man's get-togethers but this is understood and accepted. When observing a man's circle of social contacts, we can often see that the man's wife can be his primary source of support and encouragement. While this can be a wonderful thing to do, it can lead to immense problems if the wife passes away first.

When this happened with our family, Dad was at the mid-stage of Alzheimer's disease — requiring our constant prompting and reminding of things — but still aware enough of the associated facts to respond. When we had to repeatedly tell him of Mom's death, I remember how Dad was both devastated and lost. I could see his pain as he tried unsuccessfully to mask his tears. For that reason, we wondered if it was actually the proper thing to keep telling Dad the truth, but, ethically, we decided it was the only thing we could do. You may feel differently. Unfortunately, there was very little we could do for him as a family but try to provide comfort. The good thing was that Dad quickly forgot about our conversation, but we would always have to repeat this process within the next few minutes. As with the course of Alzheimer's, Dad eventually forgot his wife and no longer asked about her.

For both women and men, dealing with any negative feelings caused by caregiving is vitally important. Keeping all of this inside of you is neither effective nor realistic. While I am not a doctor, it is easy to understand how stress can affect you in many ways — physically, mentally, and emotionally. If you let stress grow, it can become unmanageable and could lead to depression or even worse.

One could potentially argue that a male caregiver may become more prone to stress by keeping quiet. The problem of caregiving can be far too big for one person to handle. Aging and the associated decline are not things we can solve. We can take various medications to cure us from ailments, but there is no pill to stop us from growing older. With having helped both of my own aging parents and experienced such problems myself, my best advice for male caregivers is to find healthy outlets and use them on a regular basis. If you're not in this category yourself, please recommend this advice to a male caregiver you know. If your words fall on deaf ears, don't be discouraged or give up but instead persist until the message gets through.

One such outlet for me proved to be a support group. After Mom and Dad both died, I attended a bereavement group and was pleased to see I was not the only man in attendance. Opening up did take some time, but I found I was encouraged to do so and sharing with others in a safe and supportive environment lifted the weight from my shoulders.

Getting some men to admit they need help may take some doing and repeated prodding. Men don't always ask for directions when traveling or read the product assembly instructions first; however, they may be more likely to listen to the advice of a family doctor who can diagnose a potential or existing problem within the privacy of an examination room and without judgment. Male caregivers can begin by booking a complete physical exam with their doctors. Complete physical exams become increasingly important for men to undergo, as they age. A doctor will be able to identify the signs of stress and recommend either a prescription or lifestyle change.

To draw an analogy, caregiving (whether undertaken by a man or a woman) can be much like driving your vehicle on a road trip. There are many roads to the same destination, which of those routes you choose will depend on your own comfort level, the amount of time you have, the number of passengers in the car and their preferences, the number of other drivers, knowledge of the route, and driving experience. If you have ever driven the Pacific Coast Highway in California, you'll know this is not the quickest road between two points but it certainly offers some exceptional scenery. Drivers are encouraged to pull over to the side of the road to snap photos and dawdle along. As a caregiver, you will slide into the driver's seat and may not necessarily know how or when you will reach your final destination. As a caregiver, how you get there is of much less consequence than what you do and how you respond along the way. Reacting to situations is a natural human response and men and women dramatically differ in this department.

In all honesty, when it comes to serving as a caregiver, it shouldn't matter which gender you are. What should take more precedence is that both men and women can effectively provide care for an aging loved one; that person's well-being will be, and should always remain, a priority. How it is accomplished will be different for everyone. The common thread is that all people will respond in some manner (either proactively or reactively) and this is what we should be looking at more carefully.

I like to think that I was just as conscientious a caregiver with my mother and father as my two sisters were. There were jobs which were better suited for me than them and vice versa. Between my two sisters and me, we each responded in our own ways, which worked well for our parents.

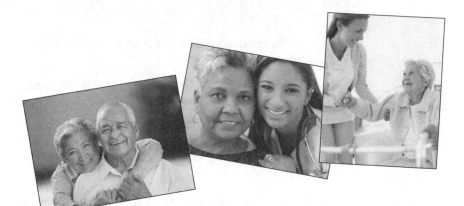

Chapter 11
Obamacare:
What It Means for Seniors
and Family Caregivers

*"The future of health-care security should include
flexibility from the federal government to allow us to
serve the state's most vulnerable citizens."*

– Thomas Vilsack

March 23, 2010, will be a date in United States history that many
Americans won't forget for some time. On this date, President
Barack Obama signed into law the *Patient Protection and Affordable
Care Act* (otherwise known as the PPACA, ACA, or "Obamacare").

The premise of Obamacare was simple — although the delivery
has proven to be very complex. It would provide an option for low-
er-income and even middle-class Americans who could not afford to
buy private health-care insurance. The concept of universal health
care in the United States has been proposed before by former Pres-
idents Theodore Roosevelt, Harry Truman, and Bill Clinton. Year

after year, however, Americans have publicly opposed the idea (disliking the idea of government-run health care).

While many Americans are still scratching their heads in confusion over the whole plan, we should remember and recognize that President Obama does have personal caregiving experience (his grandparents and his mother) and has also seen his wife, the First Lady Michelle Obama, provide care for her own father (diagnosed with Multiple Sclerosis).

As a caregiver, how does Obamacare affect you and your loved one? Granted, you will need to understand and work with the law; however, what Obamacare offers your parent (along with you), will likely be your bottom line.

As many seeking health-care insurance coverage have found, they can be refused coverage (or are charged through the roof) due to a preexisting medical condition. With Obamacare, the plan, reportedly, welcomes all individuals and the associated costs will be controlled. Many seniors have limited incomes. Considering the ever-rising costs of care, any way to reduce the expense should come as good news to seniors and their family caregivers.

Seniors on Obamacare will receive an annual complete physical exam (otherwise known as a "wellness visit"). In addition, colorectal screening and mammograms are available and, currently, are covered by the *Affordable Care Act*.

Obamacare assures a prescription drug coverage gap reduction. Before the changes, a senior on Medicare (and his or her insurance providers) paid a specified amount of money for prescription drugs. When a person reached a cap on insurance benefits, he or she would be required to pay the balance out of pocket. If a senior cannot afford to purchase prescribed medication, or attempts to stretch out a prescription to make it last longer due to this coverage gap, it is not much use.

Another promise of Obamacare is to make more information regarding nursing homes public for those on Medicare. The following includes what seniors and their families will now be able to access in regards to public information:

- Names of the owners of the facilities and the affiliated parties.
- People on the governing boards and how the organization is structured.

- Staff information for each facility (e.g., how many residents live there, hours of care per day for each resident, staff turnover, and length of staff service).

- Summary information about the number of substantiated complaints, the type of complaints, severity, and outcomes.

- Civil monetary penalties that are levied against the facility, its employees, and its contractors, or other agents.

- Any adjudicated criminal violations by the nursing facility or its employees (e.g., elder abuse violations that occur outside the facility).

1. Stay Informed

With more expected changes to be introduced in the years ahead (Obamacare is a five-year plan), it will be important for caregivers to remain educated about the Act. One method that caregivers can stay informed is by monitoring the media (e.g., television news programs, radio talk shows, newspapers, and magazine articles).

Another way for caregivers to stay current is to regularly check online at Medicare.gov. This website explains the *Affordable Care Act* in more detail as well as announces any and all changes introduced. To learn more, caregivers and seniors can call the Obamacare information hotline at 1-800-318-2596. Call-center agents will answer questions, advise on plan selection, and assist with paperwork completion.

A staff member at your local senior's association might be knowledgeable about this Act and be open to a detailed discussion; it doesn't hurt to pick up the phone, call, and ask. Although there seems to be more of a push these days towards customers accessing online information, sometimes websites are difficult to navigate (seniors may also be unfamiliar with or experience a phobia about the Internet); a face-to-face conversation can be appreciated and people can get the answers they want and/or need.

A further source of information is the American Association of Retired Persons (AARP) website where visitors can find news on Obamacare under the "Health" tab (www.aarp.org/health).

President Obama has not delayed to implement various plans to support caregivers across the country during his time in political office. These include the *Caregivers and Veterans Omnibus Health*

Services Act of 2010, the White House Middle Class Task Force Report (2010), and The National Plan to Address Alzheimer's Disease (2011). The National Plan to Address Alzheimer's Disease has caught the eye of those at the Alzheimer's Association who are publicly thankful that the Obama administration has authorized $100 million (a sizeable financial statement towards the plight of caregivers) at that time towards finding a cure for this disease and related caregiver support (www.alz.org/news_and_events_alz_association_applauds_obama_administration.asp).

It can be argued that the President certainly knows of and understands the issues caregivers experience and, judging by his actions, seems to be looking after their best interests. However this Obamacare plan turns out in the future, we cannot deny that for seniors and their family caregivers, health care is a primary concern. Whether you like the idea of Obamacare or not, one thing is for certain is that the *Affordable Care Act* is quite ambitious and complex.

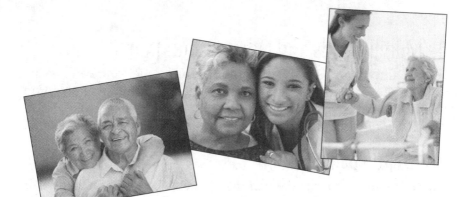

Chapter 12
Mobility Aids and
Emergency Safety Devices

"Remember, if you ever need a helping hand, it's at the end of your arm. As you get older, remember that you have another hand: The first is to help yourself, the second is to help others."

– Audrey Hepburn

This chapter will introduce you to a number of helpful mobility aids and safety products to make a senior's life easier and safer. It's important for you to purchase these items from reputable, established dealers and ensure there is a warranty or exchange program in place. With personal items, carefully consider the fit (e.g., a walker, wheelchair, scooter, or lift chair is not a "one size fits all" piece of equipment). Can your parent be sized or is the item adjustable? Of course, there are many mobility aids and other senior-friendly products on the market today, with more being routinely developed based on demand. This chapter gives you a small sampling of both large and small products that can dramatically help your parents in their daily lives.

1. Mobility Aids and Other Useful Items

Browse through a daily living store for seniors' aids and you may be amazed at what you can find. If you don't spot something, mention this to the store staff. They may be able to special order it for or serve as a direct pipeline to the manufacturers to invent a new product.

1.1 Walk-in bathtubs

These ingenious tubs make bathing a breeze for a senior. A door or sliding panel in the side of the tub can be opened by the user prior to filling the tub and taking a bath. Water pressure ensures a tight seal on the door/panel, so there is no leakage. The senior can easily step in, rather than up and over the bathtub edge, and sit down. Regular warm baths keep seniors clean (and thereby promote good health), relax arthritic bones and joints, and just feel great.

1.2 Stair lifts

A common set of stairs can become a huge obstacle for someone lacking the strength to climb them. The second floor or the basement of a home can become completely shut off because a senior may not be able to gain access.

As I witnessed with my mother, stairs into the home can also become restrictive. Consider that the entrance stairs may pose a risk; for example, not only could a senior trip and face potential injury, he or she could be trapped inside the home and unable to escape quickly in the case of a fire or other emergency.

Outside stairs also need to be shoveled clear of snow and even sanded during the winter. With a powered stair lift, your parent can smoothly ride up and down an interior or exterior staircase using a remote. A common feature on stair lifts is a battery backup; should there be a power outage, you will not want your parent to be stranded halfway between floors.

1.3 Lift chairs

Combining comfort and convenience, lift chairs make it easier for a senior to sit or stand. Your parent can simply back up into the chair and be gradually lowered into a seating position. Standing from the chair is equally easy as the user can press a button to have the chair gradually rise and tilt slightly forward. Note that with lift chairs, sizing is important — one size of chair does not fit everybody. When a person is sitting properly, his or her knees should be bent at right angles with feet flat on the floor. Lift chairs are available in an array of models and colors with various reclining positions for the comfort of the user. Your parent can sit upright, lean back to watch television, or rest flat for an afternoon nap.

1.4 Walkers

If your mother or father is not restricted to a wheelchair or bed, a walker can help with more secure standing and moving around. A walker must be sized correctly for the individual using it (Mom or Dad will have to lean forward slightly to hold on, but should remain upright when pushing the walker forward) and it will feature a hand brake to stop this mobility aid from dangerously rolling forward or backward without notice.

Many walkers can also be transformed into chairs, which is handy for the tiring senior to use for resting. There are also a variety of colorful and useful bags that can be attached to a walker for accessible storage.

1.5 Scooters

Scooters are mechanical devices that provide increased mobility, independence, and safety. Mobility scooters are usually powered by a rechargeable battery system and come with various options. Before purchasing a scooter, carefully consider the intended usage. Key questions to ask include the following:

- Where will the scooter be used (indoors or outdoors)?
- For what purpose will the scooter be used?
- Will the scooter be easily transportable?
- Can the scooter be easily disassembled?
- What is the maximum weight capacity of the scooter?

A three-wheeled model will be quite nimble and perfect for tight maneuvering inside a home, while a four-wheeled model is built for the outdoors and will be far more stable and rugged.

It may take some convincing on your part to encourage your parent to take a scooter for a test drive as the transition to a scooter may be viewed as completely unnecessary. While I have been remembering my father for the most part in this book, I recall when my mother finally purchased her scooter. At first she didn't want one (and fought tooth and nail before admitting such a machine could help her), but when she finally got in the driver's seat, she greatly enjoyed her enhanced independence.

With both walkers and scooters, take the time to disassemble and reassemble them at the store prior to purchase. It can be advantageous to have your parent work with the walker or scooter; take note if they have any difficulties doing so. Don't just watch the salesperson do this; because he or she may be demonstrating a product repeatedly, the process may seem smooth and easy to do, but may not be for you when you get it home.

1.6 Grab bars

Install grab bars firmly along walls, ensuring they are well within reach. Such grab bars can be placed throughout a senior's home; however, they are most frequently used in the bathroom. Grab bars can help a senior sit down and stand up from the toilet, pull himself or herself out of the bathtub, or steady himself or herself inside the shower. While towel racks mounted on bathroom walls may appear to work as grab bars, they can be pulled off easily and, therefore, make very poor and unsafe substitutes.

1.7 Grab poles

My sisters and I found an adjustable pole which we placed beside our parent's bed and braced it between the room's floor and ceiling. Mom found this useful as she was quite weak and could better pull herself out of bed in the mornings.

1.8 Reachers

Reachers are an excellent invention implementing a handheld pole with a set of moving pinchers on one end. These pinchers can be opened and closed, thus allowing the senior to grasp something off a higher shelf or just out of reach on the floor.

1.9 Faucet grippers

These enlarged covers slide over existing taps so they can turned on and off with ease, even with arthritic joints. I found a set that featured bright red and blue grippers to allow for quick and easy differentiation between hot and cold water temperatures. Even if someone had limited visibility, these vibrant colors could be seen.

1.10 Magnifying glass

Older eyes will have more difficulty reading smaller print. When shopping for a magnifying glass, choose one with a wider or heavier handle, making it easier to grasp.

There are also illuminated magnifying sheets which are large enough to place over a book page.

1.11 Large-buttoned telephone

In this day and age of slim, pocket-sized cell phones, large-buttoned telephones may look a little odd but they can be of tremendous value to seniors. The oversized buttons are much easier to see and press.

1.12 Bell

In this case, a bell is not for home decoration. A bell can be a very useful item for a senior still living at home. In times of distress, the bell can be rung and the sound can, typically, be heard throughout a home. You can place bells in various locations. To begin with, I would highly recommend placing a bell in the senior's bathroom. If you think of the emergency call buttons or pull cords in hospital bathrooms — these are installed for very good reasons.

1.13 Nonslip grip mat

Such a mat can be of tremendous value in the senior's bathroom. Wet floors from bathing or showering can prove to be highly slippery and an unsteady senior could easily fall.

1.14 Raised toilet seats

Raised toilet seats are handy for seniors who may encounter difficulties when going to the bathroom. Such seats can be either connected to the toilet base or be portable for easier storage and transport. With a brace bolted to the bathroom floor or a grab bar installed on the wall beside the toilet, your parent will always have a helping hand, even if you are not there to help.

1.15 Weighted and ergonomic cutlery

While you or I may not think twice about picking up a fork to eat our meals, seniors can fight with this seemingly simple task. Eating can become frustrating, if not impossible, and seniors may completely miss out on their meals if their hands continually shake from arthritic tremors.

Eating requires good balance and, with unsteady hands, food can continually fall from a fork or spoon. The senior can hold and use heavier cutlery with more confidence. As a result, the senior will continue receiving good nourishment and feel an increased sense of pride because he or she can feed himself or herself and not rely on caregiver assistance.

There is also a wide range of ergonomically designed forks, spoons, and knives on the market to make for easier feeding. These specially designed utensils are also good for a senior who may have use of only one hand.

1.16 Cushions

Cushions come in many shapes and sizes and also vary immensely in firmness. You can place a cushion on a senior's chair for increased comfort, use one for sleeping, or slide one into one side of a wheelchair to help prop up your parent. Check what kind of filling the cushion has if your parent has any allergies to any type of materials.

I recall Dad began to stoop more when he was standing and slouch more when he was sitting. By using a cushion, he could sit upright.

1.17 Medication reminder

A medication reminder is another very simple, yet highly effective, product. You can often find these at your local pharmacy. A medication reminder is a plastic box with individual compartments marked for each day of the week or separated into day parts (i.e., morning and evening, or breakfast, lunch, and dinner).

If you are picking up parental prescriptions from the pharmacy, you may be able to provide the medication blister packs to institution staff to split up as needed. Caregivers can separate different prescription medication and place pills in each compartment. Doing this will provide an excellent visual for your parent to take the pills. This will also be useful for any visiting caregiver if he or she will be with your parent at medication time. The caregiver can simply be directed to that specific day's pills. A medication reminder will also help you, the caregiver, to see if your parent did take the prescribed pills.

1.18 Pill crusher

Depending on your parent's health needs, a good-sized handful of medications may be prescribed. That handful of pills, both in quantity and in potential size, may be difficult to ingest. With a pill crusher, medication can be split up into easier-to-swallow powder. If a parent refuses to take his or her medication for any reason, try disguising it. While Dad would sometimes resist taking a pill or two, he would never refuse a bowl of ice cream (in which medication powder could be sprinkled and cleverly disguised).

1.19 Wall calendar

Hang a wall calendar in a conspicuous spot where your parent can easily see it. I like the "monthly calendar" format rather than a day planner because it can better show scheduled appointments ahead of time.

Your wall calendar should feature large enough date squares to allow room for multiple appointments on a single day. One idea which could work for you is to color-code the scheduled appointments. Write down the important doctor's appointment in red ink, the weekly church visit in blue ink, and other intermittent events in black ink. Use darker ink to make things easier to read.

Instead of a wall calendar, you could also use a small whiteboard, where you could list upcoming appointments along with accompanying pick-up times so your parent will know when you will arrive.

2. Emergency Safety Devices

There are numerous safety and security products available for seniors. Note that with any type of alarm system, be cognizant of how the alert is sounded. For example, a flashing light corresponding to a room number may be temporarily overlooked by a nurse distracted with another resident. Therefore, it could be wise to look at both auditory and visual alarms.

2.1 Personal security alarms

Typically worn around the neck as a pendant, personal security alarms are commonly patched directly through to an around-the-clock call center. Watchful staff can immediately notify you, call the senior's neighbors, or dispatch an ambulance to the senior's residence.

2.2 MedicAlert bracelets

Providing fashion and functionality, attractive MedicAlert bracelets can be engraved with a senior's health records, allergies, or current diagnosis. Should a senior require immediate care, proper help will be provided without lengthy delays. For your parent's comfort, choose a MedicAlert that fits well around your parent's wrist and one that will not irritate his or her skin.

2.3 Emergency telephone call buttons

Emergency telephone call buttons are often programmed to reach the facility's front office or nursing station. By pushing one button (rather than dialing multiple numbers), an alert will be sounded and help can arrive quickly. While the one-button operation provides ease of use for a senior in need, the telephone must be within easy reach for the button to be most effective.

3. Travel Kit

Caregivers will benefit by being prepared in the sake of an emergency. One easy way to do this is to pack a small bag to carry with you when accompanying your parent to the hospital. Hospital visits can be long, drawn out, and painful experiences and caregivers can better help themselves by ensuring they have the necessary supplies. Your emergency travel kit can be kept right by your home's front door or in your vehicle and ready to grab at a moment's notice. The following are a few suggestions of items to include in your kit:

- Medical information: The doctor may not have a complete file on your parent so it's handy to have the information with you. Record and retain important personal data like your parent's birth date, birth place, medical history (independent and family), dates of surgeries and/or dental work, allergies, current medications and dosages as well as other doctor's names and contact information. (You can complete the medical worksheets 7 and 8 included in the download kit and keep these in your travel kit.)

- Book: This can help while away the time waiting to see or hear from a doctor.

- Puzzle book: If you're not a reader, include a book of puzzles or word searches to use while waiting. Remember to pack a pencil and eraser as well.

- Clothes: A change of clothes for both you and/or your loved one can be beneficial. After spending some time in a hospital, a clean shirt and socks for both of you will be greatly appreciated.

- Notepad and pens: You'll likely hear some news and/or recommendations from your loved one's doctor. Recording this information on paper will help you remember.

- Snacks: The hospital cafeteria may not be open when you visit and there are no guarantees as to what you may find for food in hospital vending machines. Granola bars, packaged nuts, raisins, and dried fruit are good snacks for caregivers as they are healthy, nourishing, and have a longer shelf life than many other foods. Chocolate may be tempting, but it could melt inside of your bag. Sugar-free candies can also be a good option.

- Water bottle: To reduce possible spillage inside your bag, tuck an empty water bottle inside. You can fill it from a water fountain or in a hospital restroom when you arrive.

- Small toilet kit: You won't get the luxury of a shower or bath while at the hospital, but you can feel and look better by packing along a toothbrush, toothpaste, a small bottle of mouthwash, disposable razor, shaving cream, hand lotion, lip balm, deodorant, nail clippers, nail file, and makeup.

- Spare change: If you can't use your cell phone inside the hospital (due to possible interference with medical equipment) and you need to make a call, you may be able to use a public pay phone. You might also need some spare change to feed a parking meter.

- MP3 player, iPod, or tablet: Load up your music device with a few of your favorite songs and then slide on the headphones. In addition to passing the time, music can also soothe you in a potentially stressful situation of not knowing about your loved one's health. Caregivers visiting the hospital can also while away the hours by watching movies on a tablet.

- Cell phone charging cord: If you've ever had your cell phone fail on you, you know how frustrating it can be. Caregivers may need to quickly connect with other family members and by having an extra charging cord along will ensure that you can use your phone if, and when, you need to.

These are just a few recommendations for your own caregiver's hospital emergency bag; you can customize the contents to your needs.

Should you ever need to go rushing off to the hospital, don't forget any pets owned by either you or your parent. Animals will have needs when either of you is away; please leave them extra food and water or arrange for a friend to come visit and tend to the pets if you expect to be away for an extended period of time. On the chance that Mom or Dad may have an accident and require an ambulance before you can arrive, a card reading something like "I Have a Pet Still at Home" in a parental purse or wallet can alert hospital staff of an animal that may be in distress and require attention.

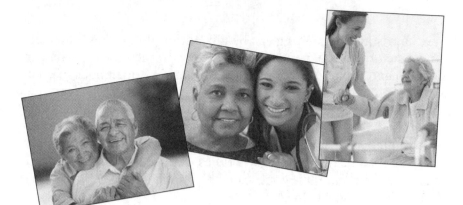

Chapter 13
Finding Joy in Caregiving

"What seems to us as bitter trials are often blessings in disguise."

– Oscar Wilde

Caring for both my mother and father were some of the hardest things I ever had to do; I was neither expecting nor prepared for this role. Watching a parent decline without being able to stop the process can be a very complicated matter. Personally, I helplessly witnessed many changes in my father; certainly one of the most apparent was the complete loss of his mental faculties. Dad, once an avid book lover, was reduced to being barely able to clutch a book in his hands, and with only the faintest recognition.

No matter what health condition you are dealing with, you too can expect a difficult journey. Caregiving can be trying because you can be torn physically, mentally, and emotionally in many different directions, simultaneously. You may be stretched to your very limits and then even past these limits. As a caregiver, you may find there are not enough hours in the day or days in the week to accomplish everything that needs to be done. As a caregiver, you may be run ragged trying to balance everything, but you will need to endure.

Surprisingly, caregiving can be a beautiful thing. This may seem contradictory to you, yet during these most difficult times, you can develop and forge stronger family relationships, open lines of communication between parents and siblings, become better organized, and strengthen your own personal resolve. Like a needle in a haystack, these joyous times in caregiving may be difficult to find. When preoccupied with tending to your parent's immediate needs, you may not even recognize the good times until years later — perhaps even after your parent is gone. You can consider these hidden gems that you will fondly hold close.

I do not believe that caregiving is either burdensome or obligatory. You are simply returning the favor to your parents who tended to you as a growing child. A common feeling amongst caregivers is that it is now "their turn." When approaching this role properly, you will find your own inner strengths and survive because doing this will make you a stronger, more confident, mature, compassionate, better, and wiser person. Whether it is through the touch of your parent's hand, a soft kiss, a smile, a warm hug, another expression of love, or a confession made, you may find moments which move you or draw you much closer to your mother or father. While I lost my father twice (once when he forgot who I was and again when he passed away), I also gained a father I never truly knew.

To further explain, my father was always an intensely private man. I never really knew him. I only grasped this fact in his later years when I finally began to understand his nature. As a result of Alzheimer's disease, Dad was unable to hide behind his emotionally protective wall any longer and his true personality and characteristics emerged. I could better see who Dad was as his wall crumbled. The cards that Dad had been dealt in life became far more apparent. As an only child, Dad looked to his parents for love and support. My grandfather died when Dad was quite young, leaving only him as a small boy, and his mother. Therefore, without that father figure of his own, Dad had no role model to follow.

I am not a parent myself but I recognize that much of parenting is learning as one goes, which is very similar to caregiving. Mirroring one's own experience can be very helpful. Dad had no such experience but was the best father he could be, given what he had. Due to his Alzheimer's disease, this aging man became a fun-loving child — a child with a kind, gentle soul who liked to be hugged. Although

Dad could not remember, he remained a human being, deserving of the utmost respect, care, quality of life, love, and dignity.

With joy comes laughter. Although caregiving is a serious matter, please allow yourself to laugh. When only visiting my mother, she slipped and fell on the floor. Concerned, I immediately rushed to her, and, much to my surprise, she started laughing! Mom always had a quirky sense of humor. Thankfully, she was absolutely fine. She explained that her reason for laughing was because she felt like an overturned turtle, too weak to right herself or stand up again. To emphasize her point, Mom ineffectively weakly waved her arms and legs in the air. Greatly relieved, I laughed with her, extended my hand, and helped her to her feet. As a caregiver, you will have tremendous responsibility on your shoulders, but this does not mean that you must be serious at all times.

There are many other joys involved with caregiving. You will increase your opportunities for self-discovery. Although your learning curve may be steep, you will learn about your parent's medical condition as well as your own abilities. Always remember, you can succeed.

You will discover who your true friends are. These friends will be the ones who will continually support, encourage, and listen to you — all the time without judgment. These friends will not only offer to help you in whatever way they can, they will follow through on those commitments.

You will become better organized. There is nothing like minding your parent's matters to teach you improved organizational skills. If you have not done so already, caregiving can also remind you to get your own affairs in order. Have you drafted up your own will?

You will be far happier if you remain easy on yourself. Listen to your own body; it will tell you when you are doing too much. It is up to you to acknowledge those messages. You are only one person and, for this reason alone, it is imperative for you to seek caregiving help and to take your own personal respite time. Practicing self-care is not selfish! It is not my intention to preach but only to advise and guide you as you look ahead. Knowing everything that lies ahead for you as a caregiver is impossible, but you can begin to prepare yourself.

One of the best things you can do for yourself and your loved one is to accept. Accept your own limitations. Accept what you cannot change. Accept the fact that everybody makes mistakes — we are not perfect, nor can we ever be perfect. Accept and recognize your own human restrictions. You may want to try to accomplish all which needs to be done yourself (or mistakenly believe that doing so is possible); however, this is simply not realistic.

You must also accept time limitations. There are only 24 hours in a day. With eight hours required for a good night's sleep and eight hours on the job, two-thirds of your day are already spoken for. In the remaining time, you must juggle many other responsibilities including your own family, housework, and shopping. Don't try to fool yourself that you can multitask successfully; the more you take on, the less you are likely to accomplish and/or complete. Don't short-change yourself on sleep to give yourself more time in the day.

Accept the cards you have been dealt in life. While you may feel you have been given a terrible hand, these same cards can offer many other rewards — both large and small.

Congratulate yourself on a daily basis for what you do and can do. Not everybody can, or will become a caregiver. You have chosen this path and committed to see the job through to the end. Not everybody has the fortitude to do this and you are to be admired and appreciated.

While I have tried to provide directions and well-meant advice to you, I admittedly do not have all the answers. A guidebook such as this can provide a general idea of how to deal with your situation. There is no complete caregiving map or any directional road signs, because each tool would be inadequate — each caregiver's starting points, routes traveled, and final destinations vary. Each caregiver can be vastly different as well. With that said, you will also find similarities between caregivers' personal stories, which include both tragedies and triumphs.

If I said that caregiving was easy, it would be an outright lie. You can, however, take the steps to make the job easier. Good luck and best wishes on your own caregiving journey. Make yourself and your parents proud!

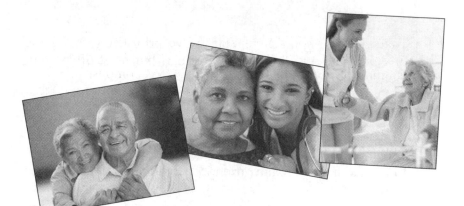

Chapter 14
Final Thoughts

"Final thoughts are so, you know, final. Let's call them closing words."

– Craig Armstrong

While this book is now coming to a close, know that your own caregiving journey is just beginning. Your parent will develop as the lead character and you will serve in a supporting role. Your own storyline will unfold as you fulfill your various caregiving responsibilities. There are an unknown number of chapters ahead of you and your outcome cannot be completely certain (there may well be a plot twist or two before you finish); however, you will learn, manage, grow stronger, and experience both joy and sorrow.

If you find yourself questioning yourself as a caregiver (asking questions like "Am I doing enough?" "Am I making the right decisions?" "Would this be what Mom and Dad wants?"), know this is to be expected – being human you can only do so much. When you feel self-doubt creeping in or lingering with you, glance through the following words of advice. I have listed these in bullet form to provide you with a quick and easy read.

- Take time for yourself regularly. I've prioritized this as the first point because it is very important but most often completely overlooked by caregivers.
- Know that you are never alone as a caregiver.
- Prepare for the future.
- Remain flexible with your time.
- Enlist the help of family, friends, neighbors, and health-care workers.
- Allow others to help and accept their offers. If others are willing to help but uncertain as to how to do so, make a few recommendations (e.g. "I could use someone to drive Mom/Dad to the appointment").
- Think outside the caregiving box. Who else can help you, when, and how?
- Accept your own, and others', limitations.
- Set achievable caregiving goals.
- Trust your instincts.
- Allow yourself to cry, if need be.
- Allow yourself to laugh, when appropriate.
- Take time for yourself regularly (Yes, I have mentioned this before, but it bears repeating).
- Remember there is joy in caregiving even though it may not be immediately obvious.
- Continue to learn everything you can about your parent's health condition, the associated symptoms to watch for, the diagnosis to expect, and how you can best help as a caregiver.
- Treat your parent with respect and dignity. Despite whatever medical ailment is involved, your parent remains a human being.
- Ensure that your parent is enjoying the best quality of life possible.
- Keep your parent comfortable (cool in the summer and warm in the winter).
- Love your parent unconditionally.
- Manage your parent's affairs ethically.

- Protect your parent from possible physical, mental, emotional, and financial abuse.
- Stay strong to your beliefs.
- Take pride in what you do as a caregiver.
- Work to release of any lingering self-doubt and guilt that you are not doing enough as a caregiver.
- Exercise patience with yourself, your parent, and others.
- Value your time and efforts as a caregiver.
- Maintain open lines of communication between all parties involved. Share and listen.
- Decide what you can and cannot do as a caregiver (due to geographical or emotional distance).
- Understand that grieving a loss can begin even before death.
- Seek out caregiving coping mechanisms than can work for you. Experiment with other options to find other means of managing.
- Reflect on what is most important in your life and your parent's life.
- Ask yourself, "What would Mom or Dad do or want in this situation?"
- Strive for balance in your own personal and professional lives.
- Expect and embrace uncertainty with how to proceed with caregiving.
- Communicate with your own family.
- Dismiss self-doubt that you cannot provide adequate or quality care for your parent. Even without a related health, medical, banking, or legal background, there is much you can still do.
- Avoid sacrificing your own life for another's.
- Rest when needed.
- Explain your impending need for time away from work ahead of time. Discuss possible work arrangements including paid leave, reduced hours, or work-sharing with another individual. If you are an entrepreneur, can you give those reins to a trusted friend or colleague to help run your business on a temporary basis?

- Lobby politicians for increased caregiving funding, tax breaks, and service or support programs at civic, state, and national levels.

- Again, take time for yourself regularly. Please do not forget your own needs.

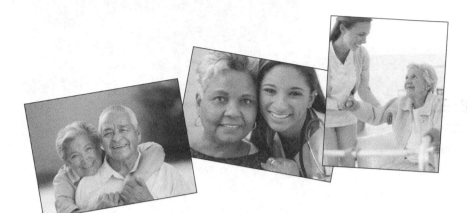

Download kit

Please enter the URL you see in the box below into your computer web browser to access and download the kit.

www.self-counsel.com/updates/successfulcaregiver/15kit.htm

The download kit offers forms in MS Word and/or PDF format so you can edit as needed. It includes:

- Worksheets to help you keep track of caregiving needs.
- Online resources.

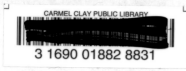

CARMEL CLAY PUBLIC LIBRARY

3 1690 01882 8831

CARMEL CLAY PUBLIC LIBRARY
Renewal Line: (317) 814-3936
www.carmel.lib.in.us

WITHDRAWN FROM
CARMEL CLAY
PUBLIC LIBRARY